T0201912

Standards for the Management of Open Fractures

Standards for the Management of Open Fractures

Edited by

Simon Eccles, Bob Handley, Umraz Khan,
Iain McFadyen, Jagdeep Nanchahal,
Selvadurai Nayagam
(listed alphabetically)

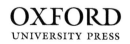

OXFORD
UNIVERSITY PRESS

Great Clarendon Street, Oxford, OX2 6DP,
United Kingdom

Oxford University Press is a department of the University of Oxford.
It furthers the University's objective of excellence in research, scholarship,
and education by publishing worldwide. Oxford is a registered trade mark of
Oxford University Press in the UK and in certain other countries

© BAPRAS and BOA 2020

The moral rights of the authors have been asserted

Impression: 1

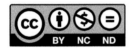
Published in the United States of America by Oxford University Press
198 Madison Avenue, New York, NY 10016, United States of America

British Library Cataloguing in Publication Data

Data available

Library of Congress Control Number: 2020935855

ISBN 978–0–19–884936–0

Printed and bound by
CPI Group (UK) Ltd, Croydon, CR0 4YY

Foreword

Our understanding of trauma pathology, the effectiveness of interventions, and tissue recovery continue to improve. Much has changed in the system of trauma care in recent years in Britain; we have sadly also learnt from war zones and terrorism at home. A step change has been the improvement in the quality of our approach to research and the resultant evidence. It is therefore wholly appropriate, and I am delighted to see, that such new learning and treatment opportunities are central to the refreshing of these important standards for the management of open fractures. Their value lies now in their dissemination and adoption; I commend this book to all practising orthopaedic trauma and plastic surgeons.

Keith Willett
Medical Director for Acute Care, NHS England
National Director for Emergency Preparedness, NHS England

Preface

The first edition of the British Association of Plastic, Reconstructive and Aesthetic Surgeons (BAPRAS) and British Orthopaedic Association (BOA) book *Severe Open Fractures of the Lower Limb* in 2009 set the standards for collaborative management of these injuries. There have subsequently been major advances in the logistics, the provision, and the monitoring of care for patients sustaining injuries with open fractures in the UK. In 2012 major trauma centres and networks were established across England, in 2016 the National Institute for Health and Care Excellence (NICE) published guidance for managing complex fractures, and in 2017 based on this the Open Fracture BOAST (BOA STandards) from the British Orthopaedic Association was updated.

In the light of these changes a new edition of this book was needed. As an example of orthoplastic collaboration the opportunity was taken to expand on this work and involve a broader group in its production on behalf of BAPRAS and the BOA. We have been able to draw on the expertise of many colleagues with great experience and in-depth knowledge of managing these injuries. The contents have been updated to reflect the recent NICE Guidelines and latest literature. Paradigms in management have been generated through an evidence base and, when a clear choice between available alternatives for management is absent, the contributors provide a balanced view by highlighting the relative merits and drawbacks of each. In addition to the evidence-based recommendations, the authors have provided technical tips and descriptions of 'how to do it' where relevant.

The NICE Guidelines 2016 and the Open Fracture BOAST 2017 consolidated the orthoplastic approach to open fractures advocated in the first edition of this book. In each of those guidelines the range of injuries included was extended beyond the lower limb, hence this book now being titled *Open Fracture Standards* to accommodate this. It remains the case that much of the evidence and consequently the narrative of this book refers to the tibia. The book has been expanded to include new topics of relevance to the patient with open fractures. There are now chapters on how to set up a service to deal with open fractures, the psychological aspects of trauma, and management of fractures in the young and elderly populations. However, the core message and express intent is to enable the orthoplastic management of an open fracture whenever required. We envisage that this new edition with the included NICE Guidelines and Open

Fracture BOAST will provide an easily accessible source of the guidance and standards for management of patients with open fractures.

We made the decision that in this publication we would replace the term **debridement** with the term **wound excision,** both in our own narrative and when referring to the publications of others. This should lead the reader to the principle that successful separation of tissues that are contaminated or non-viable from those that are healthy and viable relies on surgical excision of the former. Surgical access to the area requiring excision will include an extension of the traumatic wound by incision. The change in terminology from **debridement** to **wound excision** then encourages the concept that completion of the process relies on more than just lavage and dilution of contaminants.

Acknowledgements

BAPRAS and BOA are grateful to the following for each making an unrestricted educational grant to defray the costs of publication and thus allowing the Standards to be made available more widely. The grants had no influence on the content of the book.

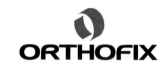

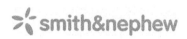

Contents

Contributors

A central theme of this book is collaboration. It is itself a manifestation of an orthoplastic team working to a common purpose. Its strength comes from the group responsibility taken for the efforts of the individual contributors; hence an absence of names on the front cover and at the beginning of chapters. While all the authors were able to review, discuss, and agree every chapter to broaden the review of the evidence, there were lead contributors to each chapter who did significant work that should be recognized. Listed below are the contributors to this book in alphabetical order. By each name is noted the chapter numbers where they were a lead author; additionally if they were involved in producing the relevant NICE Complex Fracture Guidelines or on the BOA Trauma group (the origin of the Open Fracture BOAST).

Alexander Aquilina, BSc, MB ChB, MRCS, MSc
Clinical Research Fellow and DPhil candidate
Oxford Trauma Group
Nuffield Department of Orthopaedics, Rheumatology and Musculoskeletal
   Sciences
University of Oxford
Chapter 16

Bridget L. Atkins, MSc, FRCP, FRCPath
Consultant in Infectious Diseases and Microbiology
Oxford University Hospitals NHS Foundation Trust
Honorary Senior Lecturer, University of Oxford
Chapter 1

Deepa Bose, MBBS, FRCS(Tr&Orth)
Consultant in Orthopaedic Trauma and Limb Reconstruction
Queen Elizabeth Hospital Birmingham
Chapter 9

*Simon Britten, BM, LLM, FRCS(Eng), FRCS(Tr&Orth)
Consultant Trauma and Orthopaedic Surgeon
Leeds Teaching Hospitals
Honorary Senior Lecturer, University of Leeds
Secretary British Limb Reconstruction Society

Cherylene Camps, MSc, MC Para
Clinical Development Lead
East Midlands Ambulance Service NHS Trust
HEMS/Critical Care Paramedic
The Air Ambulance Service
Associate Lecturer Paramedic Science Practice, Sheffield Hallam University
Contributor JRCALC Limb Trauma
Member NICE Guidance Development Groups Complex Fractures
Chapter 1

James K.-K. Chan, MA, DPhil, FRCS(Plast)
Consultant in Plastic Reconstructive Surgery
Stoke Mandeville Hospital, Buckinghamshire Healthcare NHS Trust
Honorary Departmental Clinical Lecturer, Nuffield Department of
   Orthopaedics, Rheumatology and Musculoskeletal Sciences, University of
   Oxford
Chapters 4, 7, 8

*Matthew L. Costa, FRCS(Tr&Orth), PhD
Professor of Orthopaedic Trauma Surgery
Oxford Trauma, University of Oxford
Nuffield Department of Orthopaedics, Rheumatology and Musculoskeletal
   Sciences, Oxford Trauma, Kadoorie Centre, University of Oxford
Member NICE Guidance Development Groups Complex and Non-Complex
   Fractures
Member BOA Trauma Group
Chapters 1, 5, 15, 17

*Simon Eccles, BDS, FRCS, FRCS(Plast)
Consultant Craniofacial Plastic Surgeon
Chelsea and Westminster Hospital NHS Foundation Trust
Honorary Secretary BAPRAS
Co-Chair Committee Open Fracture Standards

Miguel A. Fernandez, MBBS, MRCS, PhD

Clinical Research Fellow
Oxford Trauma
Nuffield Department of Orthopaedics, Rheumatology and Musculoskeletal
Sciences
University of Oxford
Specialty Registrar Trauma and Orthopaedic Surgery, University Hospitals
Coventry and Warwickshire NHS Trust
Chapter 15

Matthew D. Gardiner, MA, PhD, FRCS(Plast)

Consultant Hand and Plastic Surgeon
Wexham Park Hospital, Frimley Park NHS Foundation Trust
Honorary Departmental Clinical Lecturer in Plastic and Reconstructive
Surgery
Kennedy Institute of Rheumatology
Nuffield Department of Orthopaedics, Rheumatology and Musculoskeletal
Sciences
University of Oxford
Chapters 2, 3

*Victoria Giblin, MB BCh, MA(Cantab), PhD, FRCS(Plast)

Consultant in Plastic and Reconstructive Surgery
Plastics Trauma Lead Sheffield MTC
Plastics Research Lead
Northern General Hospital, Sheffield Teaching Hospitals NHS
Foundation Trust

Graeme E. Glass, PhD, FRCS(Plast)

Attending Plastic and Craniofacial Surgeon
Department of Surgery
Sidra Medicine
Doha, State of Qatar
Associate Professor of Plastic Surgery
Weill Cornell Medical College, Qatar
Chapter 10

*Xavier L. Griffin, PhD, FRCS(Tr&Orth)

Associate Professor of Trauma Surgery
Kadoorie Critical Care Research and Education Centre
Nuffield Department of Orthopaedics, Rheumatology and Musculoskeletal
    Sciences
University of Oxford
Honorary Consultant, Oxford University Hospitals NHS Foundation Trust
Deputy Co-ordinating Editor, Cochrane Bone, Joint and Muscle Trauma Group
Chapter 16

*Robert Handley, BSc, MB ChB, FRCS

Consultant Trauma and Orthopaedic Surgeon
Oxford University Hospitals NHS Foundation Trust
Vice President British Orthopaedic Association
Chair BOA Trauma Committee
National Clinical Lead GIRFT Orthopaedic Trauma
Co-chair NICE Guidance Development Groups Complex and Non-Complex
Fractures
Co-chair Open Fracture Standards Committee

*Lorraine (Loz) Harry, PhD, FRCS(Plast), MA(Cantab)

Consultant Orthoplastic Surgeon
Queen Victoria Hospital NHS Foundation Trust, East Grinstead
Brighton and Sussex University Hospitals Trust
Chapter 20

Paul Harwood, MB ChB, MSc, PGCCE, FHEA, FRCS(Tr&Orth)

Consultant Trauma and Orthopaedic Surgeon
Leeds Major Trauma Centre and Limb Reconstruction Unit
Honorary Senior Lecturer, Leeds University Medical School
Deputy Training Program Director, Trauma and Orthopaedics HEEY&H
Chapter 8

*Shehan Hettiaratchy, MA(Oxon), DM, FRCS(Plast), RAMC

Lead Surgeon and Major Trauma Director
Imperial College Healthcare NHS Trust
Honorary Clinical Senior Lecturer, Imperial College
Chapter 19

Alan Kay, FRCS, FRCS(Plast), L/RAMC
Consultant Plastic Surgeon
Royal Centre for Defence Medicine
Chapter 19

David J. Keene, DPhil, MCSP
NDORMS Research Fellow in Trauma Rehabilitation/NIHR Postdoctoral
Research Fellow
Kadoorie Centre for Critical Care Research and Education
Nuffield Department of Orthopaedics, Rheumatology and Musculoskeletal
    Sciences
University of Oxford
Chapter 16

***Umraz Khan, FCPS(Hon), FRCS(Plast)**
Head of Orthoplastics
North Bristol NHS Trust
BAPRAS Council Member
Chapters 18, 20

Graham Lawton, BSc, DMCC, MD, FRCS(Plast), RAMC
Consultant Plastic Surgeon
Imperial College Healthcare NHS Trust
Honorary Clinical Senior Lecturer, Imperial College
Senior Lecturer, Academic Department Military Surgery and Trauma, Royal
    Centre for Defence Medicine
Chapter 19

James Masters, BSc, MRCS(Eng)
Clinical Research Fellow
Oxford Trauma Group
Nuffield Department of Orthopaedics, Rheumatology and Musculoskeletal
    Sciences
University of Oxford
Chapter 1

*Iain McFadyen, FRCS(Tr&Orth)

Consultant Orthopaedic Trauma Surgeon
Royal Stoke University Hospital
Co-chair NICE Guidance Development Groups Complex and Non-Complex
Fractures
Chapter 20

*Jagdeep Nanchahal, PhD, FRCS(Plast)

Professor of Hand, Plastic and Reconstructive Surgery
Kennedy Institute of Rheumatology
Nuffield Department of Orthopaedics, Rheumatology and Musculoskeletal
Sciences
University of Oxford
Honorary Consultant, Oxford University Hospitals NHS Foundation Trust
Member NICE Guidance Development Groups Complex and Non-Complex
Fractures
Chapters 1, 2, 3, 4, 5, 7, 8, 10, 15

*Selvadurai Nayagam, BSc, MCh(Orth), FRCS(Tr&Orth)

Honorary Reader, University of Liverpool
Consultant Orthopaedic Surgeon, Royal Liverpool and Broadgreen University
and Royal Liverpool Children's NHS Trusts
Member NICE Guidance Development Groups Complex and Non-Complex
Fractures
Chapters 6, 11, 14

*Michael F. Pearse, FRCS(Tr&Orth)

Senior Clinical Lecturer, Imperial College
Consultant Orthopaedic Surgeon, Imperial Healthcare NHS Trust, St Mary's
Hospital, London
Chapters 3, 12, 13

Jowan Penn-Barwell, MB ChB, MSc, FRCS(Tr&Orth)

Consultant Orthopaedic Trauma Surgeon
Royal Navy and Oxford University Hospitals NHS Foundation Trust
Chapters 18, 19

Louise May Quarmby, MA(Hons), PGDipPsych, DClinPsy
Principal Clinical Psychologist
Oxford Major Trauma Centre
Russell Cairns Unit
John Radcliffe Hospital, Oxford
Chapter 17

*Simon Royston, MB ChB, FRCS(Tr&Orth)
Consultant Trauma and Orthopaedic Surgeon
Northern General Hospital, Sheffield

Elizabeth Tutton, PhD, RN
Senior Research Fellow
Warwick Research in Nursing
Warwick Medical School
University of Warwick
Kadoorie Critical Care Research and Education Centre
John Radcliffe Hospital, Oxford
Chapter 17

*David Wallace, BSc, MBBS, MSc, DIC, FRCS(Plast)
Consultant Plastic and Reconstructive Surgery
University Hospitals Coventry and Warwickshire

*Robert Winterton, MBBS, BMedSci, MPhil, FRCS(Plast), DipHandSurg
Consultant Plastic and Reconstructive Surgeon
Wythenshawe Hospital
Manchester University Foundation Trust

*Member of committee representing the British Association of Plastic, Reconstructive and Aesthetic Surgeons, British Orthopaedic Association, British Limb Reconstruction Society, and Orthopaedic Trauma Society, which oversaw the writing and production of these Standards.

List of Abbreviations

ABPI	ankle-brachial pressure index		FDA	Food and Drug Administration
ATLS	advanced trauma life support		LEAP	Lower Extremity Assessment Project
BAPRAS	British Association of Plastic, Reconstructive and Aesthetic Surgeons		MDT	multidisciplinary team
			MSC	mesenchymal stem cell
BMAC	Bone marrow aspirate concentrate		NICE	National Institute for Health and Care Excellence
BMP	bone morphogenetic protein		NPWT	negative pressure wound therapy
BOA	British Orthopaedic Association		OMI	outcome measurement instrument
BOAST	British Orthopaedic Association Standards for Trauma and Orthopaedics		PMMA	polymethylmethacrylate
			PRP	platelet-rich plasma
CABCDE	Circulation (exsanguinating haemorrhage), Airway, Breathing, Circulation, Disability, Exposure		PU	polyurethane
			RIA	reamer irrigator aspirator
			SF-36	Short Form 36
			SIP	Sickness Impact Profile
CDC	Centers for Disease Control		SPECT	single-photon emission computed tomography
CT	computed tomography		SSI	surgical site infection
DO	distraction osteogenesis		TARN	Trauma Audit and Research Network
EQ-5D-5L	EuroQol-Five Dimensions-Five Levels		WHIST	wound healing in surgical trauma
IV	intravenous			
ISS	Injury Severity Score			

Introduction

The management of patients suffering from trauma has advanced rapidly over the past 10 years and it is now accepted that patients with open fractures are best treated jointly by orthopaedic and plastic surgeons working together in specialist and major trauma centres. The importance of this collaborative working is reflected in the Quality Statement published by the National Institute for Health and Care Excellence (NICE) in March 2018 (NICE Quality Standard QS166 for Trauma, https://www.nice.org.uk/guidance/qs166/chapter/Quality-statement-3-Open-fractures#quality-statement-3), which states:

> People with open fractures of long bones, the hindfoot or midfoot have fixation and definitive soft tissue coverage within 72 hours of the injury if this cannot be performed at the same time as the debridement.

NICE further recognised that for collaborative management to be attainable requires not just the desire to collaborate but the appropriate infrastructure to be in place. The NICE Complex Fracture Guidelines 2016 defined an orthoplastic centre, which has the following key characteristics:

- A combined service of orthopaedic and plastic surgery consultants.
- Sufficient combined operating lists with consultants from both specialties to meet the standards for timely management of open fractures.
- Scheduled, combined review clinics for severe open fractures.
- Specialist nursing teams able to care for both fractures and flaps.

In addition, an effective orthoplastic service will also:

- Submit data on each patient to the Trauma Audit and Research Network (TARN).
- Hold regular clinical audit meetings with both orthopaedic and plastic surgeons present.

For the past 20 years the British Orthopaedic Association (BOA) and British Association of Plastic, Reconstructive and Aesthetic Surgeons (BAPRAS) have worked together to produce professional guidelines for the management of severe open tibial fractures, promoting a joint 'orthoplastics' approach to care, and this has led to the development of clinical audit standards that have been used both nationally and internationally to improve the care of trauma patients. This book reflects the new NICE guidance and builds on previous work to provide a practical guide based on the available evidence and experience of the authors. The guide covers the entire patient pathway from emergency management through to definitive care and then rehabilitation and psychosocial care. It is essential reading for all orthopaedic and plastic surgeons who manage trauma.

Professor Chris Moran
National Clinical Director for Trauma NHS-England

British Orthopaedic
Association

BRITISH ORTHOPAEDIC ASSOCIATION AND BRITISH ASSOCIATION OF PLASTIC, RECONSTRUCTIVE AND AESTHETIC SURGEONS
AUDIT STANDARDS FOR TRAUMA

BAPRAS
British Association of Plastic
Reconstructive and Aesthetic Surgeons

British Limb Reconstruction Society

OPEN FRACTURES
December 2017

Background and justification

Open fractures may require timely multidisciplinary management. The consequences of infection can be great both for the individual patient and the community. Trauma networks and hospitals require the appropriate pathways and infrastructure to manage these patients, to enable optimum recovery and to minimise the risk of infection.

Inclusions: All patients with open fractures of long bones, hind foot, or midfoot (excluding hand, wrist, forefoot or digit).

Standards for practice audit:

1. Patients with open fractures of long bones, hind foot, or midfoot should be taken directly or transferred to a specialist centre that can provide Orthoplastic* care. Patients with hand, wrist, forefoot, or digit injuries may be managed locally following similar principles.

2. Intravenous prophylactic antibiotics should be administered as soon as possible, ideally within 1 hour of injury.

3. There should be a readily accessible published network guideline for the use of antibiotics in open fractures.

4. The examination of the injured limb should include assessment and documentation of the vascular and neurological status. This should be repeated systematically, particularly after reduction manoeuvres or the application of splints. Management of suspected compartment syndrome should follow BOAST guidelines.

5. The limb should be re-aligned and splinted.

6. Patients presenting with arterial injuries in association with their fracture should be treated in accordance with the BOAST for arterial injuries.

7. In patients where an initial 'Trauma CT' is indicated there should be protocols to maximise the useful information and minimise delay:

   - The initial sequence should include a head to toes scanogram. This should be used with clinical correlation to direct further specific limb sequences during that initial CT examination.

   - There should be a local policy on the inclusion of angiography in any extremity CT related to open fractures.

8. Prior to formal debridement the wound should be handled only to remove gross contamination and to allow photography, then dressed with a saline-soaked gauze and covered with an occlusive film. 'Mini-washouts' outside the operating theatre environment are not indicated.

9. All trauma networks must have information governance policies in place that enable staff to take, use, and store photographs of open fracture wounds for clinical decision-making 24 hours a day.

10. Photographs of open fracture wounds should be taken when they are first exposed for clinical care, before debridement and at other key stages of management. These should be kept in the patient's records.

11. The formation of the management plan for fixation and coverage of open fractures and surgery for initial debridement should be undertaken concurrently by consultants in orthopaedic and plastic surgery (a combined orthoplastic approach).

12. Debridement should be performed using fasciotomy lines for wound extension where possible (see overleaf for recommended incisions for fasciotomies of the leg):

    - Immediately for highly contaminated wounds (agricultural, aquatic, sewage) or when there is an associated vascular compromise (compartment syndrome or arterial disruption producing ischaemia).

    - Within 12 hours of injury for other solitary high energy open fractures—within 24 hours of injury for all other low energy open fractures.

13. Once debridement is complete any further procedures carried out at that same sitting should be regarded as clean surgery; i.e. there should be fresh instruments and a re-prep and drape of the limb before proceeding.

14. Definitive soft tissue closure or coverage should be achieved within 72 hours of injury if it cannot be performed at the time of debridement.

15. Definitive internal stabilisation should only be carried out when it can be immediately followed with definitive soft tissue cover.

16. When a decision whether to perform limb salvage or delayed primary amputation is indicated, this should be based on a multidisciplinary assessment involving an orthopaedic surgeon, a plastic surgeon, a rehabilitation specialist, the patient and their family or carers.

17. When indicated, a delayed primary amputation should be performed within 72 hours of injury.

18. Each trauma network should submit appropriate data to the TARN, monitor its performance against national standards and audit its outcomes.

19. All patients should receive information regarding expected functional recovery and rehabilitation, including advice about return to normal activities such as work and driving.

* Orthoplastic unit: A hospital with a dedicated, combined service for orthopaedic and plastic surgery in which consultants from both specialties work simultaneously to treat open fractures as part of regular, scheduled, combined orthopaedic and plastic surgery operating lists. The surgical service is supported by combined review clinics and specialist nursing teams (from NICE guidelines).

Evidence base

NICE Complex fracture guideline https://www.nice.org.uk/guidance/ NG37/chapter/recommendations

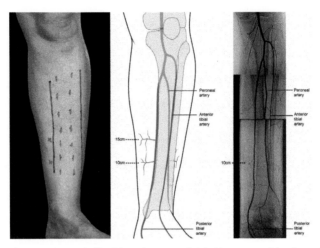

Figure showing recommended incisions for wound debridement and fasciotomies in the leg. The medical incision alone is usually sufficient for debridement and preserves the perforators arising from the posterior tibial vessels, which form the basis of local fasciocutanoeus flaps. It also provides access to the posterior tibial artery and venae commitans when required as recipient vessels for free flaps. The lateral incision is used for decompression of the anterior and peroneal compartments in patients with compartment syndrome. (A) Margins of subcutaneous border of the tibia marked in green, access incisions marked in blue and perforators arising from the medical side as red crosses. (B) Line drawing depicting the location of the perforators, with approximate indicative distances from the tip of the medical malleolus. (C) Montage of arteriogram.

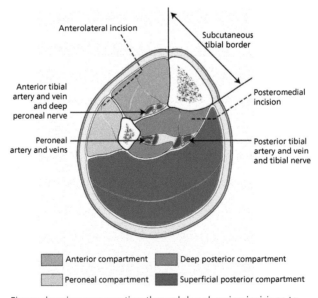

Figure showing cross section through leg showing incisions to decompress all four compartments

Chapter 1

Prehospital and Emergency Department Care, Including Prophylactic Antibiotics

Summary

1. Antibiotics should be administered intravenously as soon as an open fracture is identified, ideally within 1 hour of the injury without delaying transfer to hospital.

2. Splinting is a highly effective form of analgesia and should be performed prehospital.

3. Clinical examination of the neurological and vascular status must be thorough, performed repeatedly, and documented, particularly after an intervention has taken place.

4. Transport people with suspected open fractures directly to a major trauma centre or specialist centre that can provide orthoplastic care if a long bone, hindfoot, or midfoot are involved, or to the nearest trauma unit or emergency department if the suspected fracture is in the hand, wrist, or toes, unless there are prehospital triage indications for direct transport to a major trauma centre.

5. For isolated open fractures, orthogonal views on radiographs should be obtained. In patients where an initial 'trauma CT' (computed tomography) is indicated there should be protocols to maximise the useful information and minimise delay; the initial sequence should include a head to toes scanogram. This should be used with clinical correlation to direct further specific limb sequences during that initial CT examination.

6. There should be a local policy on the inclusion of angiography in any extremity CT related to open fractures.

7. Irrigation of the wound should not be performed prehospital or in the emergency department. It should be reserved until after surgical excision of the wound in the operating theatre.

8. Once wounds are identified they should be photographed and then covered with a saline-soaked gauze and occlusive dressing.

Prehospital

Introduction

An open long bone fracture is a serious injury not only because of the associated significant soft tissue damage but because the exposed bone is contaminated and the risk of infection increased greatly. Urgent assessment and appropriate treatment can reduce disability and improve quality of life for patients with open fractures.

Patients with open fractures should be treated in centres that can offer the full spectrum of orthoplastic services, including soft tissue and bone reconstruction. Such teams are found in major trauma centres and in some specialist orthoplastic centres. These are the preferred primary destinations for such patients (1). Although much of the evidence described here is based upon open fracture of the tibia, the principles described also apply to open fractures of other long bones, including those of the upper limb (excluding the hand and wrist), even though complex soft tissue reconstruction is required less commonly.

Not all open fractures occur in the context of high-energy trauma, but many do and a systematic approach to assess, identify, and treat the most serious injuries first is imperative. The management of the open fracture is considered concurrently with other patient co-morbidities and associated injuries. In the UK, the Major Trauma Networks have guidance based upon the international Advanced Trauma Life Support (ATLS)® system; this includes prehospital assessment, transport of patients, rapid whole-body cross-sectional imaging, and major transfusion protocols (2, 3).

Primary survey

After scene safety, the CABCDE (Circulation (exsanguinating haemorrhage), Airway, Breathing, Circulation, Disability, Exposure) principles should be followed. Although angulated fractures may draw the prehospital clinician's attention, life-threatening conditions should take priority (1–3). Exsanguinating external haemorrhage should be controlled prior to the management of airway or breathing.

Assessment of the limb

Limb assessment in the prehospital environment is dictated by the setting, other injuries, and obvious flags such as patient signs and symptoms. Once the patient's primary survey findings have been addressed, a secondary assessment of the limb can be undertaken. The paradigm of 'look, feel, and move' on limbs should identify important injuries at this stage (1), but this is omitted in the presence of obvious fractures to avoid more pain. Wounds are of relevance and raise the possibility of an open fracture. If there is doubt about an open fracture, it is safer to proceed as though open until proven otherwise; a photograph of the wound in the prehospital setting may aid decisions in treatment.

A key initial assessment is for vascular injury by the presence or absence of each of the distal pulses. Vascular deficit mandates immediate realignment. The capillary refill time can be misleading and hard signs (palpable pulses, expanding haematoma, continued bleeding) should be relied upon. Neurological assessment of motor function should test for active movements and of sensation by response to touch.

Management of limb

Adequate analgesia is important in all patients suspected of a fracture; additionally, reduction of deformity and splintage reduce bleeding and pain. If the bone ends of an open fracture retract into the wound during splinting, this information must be documented. A traction device is used if the injury is above the knee. All other long bone injuries should be splinted with a vacuum splint (1, 2). When an intervention is performed, e.g. application of a splint, the vascular and neurological assessments should be repeated and documented.

Irrigation of open fractures at the prehospital stage is not recommended but gross contamination should be removed. Clean saline-soaked gauze held with an occlusive layer should be applied to the wound. Information about potential contamination by agricultural, marine, or sewage matter needs to be relayed to the admitting team as this has direct implications for the urgency of surgical wound excision.

Antibiotics are given as soon as possible and preferably within an hour of injury. The administration of prophylactic antibiotics for patients with open fractures is supported by a Cochrane Systematic review (4), which reported an absolute risk reduction of 0.08 based on data from 913 participants in seven published studies (see the section on 'Antibiotics' for choice of antibiotics). Timing of administration of the antibiotics was found to be an independent risk factor in a retrospective study, with delay beyond 1 hour after injury associated with an increased risk of infection (odds ratio 3.78, CI 1.16–12.31) (5). The National Institute for Health and Care Excellence (NICE) recommends the administration of antibiotics within 1 hour of the injury but this should not delay transfer to hospital (4).

An elasticated field dressing may be augmented in a stepwise progression to control bleeding:

◆ direct pressure onto the wound;

◆ elevation;

◆ wound packing;

◆ prehospital tourniquet (windlass type);

◆ hospital tourniquet (pneumatic type).

The use of tourniquets or haemostatic agents should be considered only when all other methods have failed and the patient is still exsanguinating. If a tourniquet is applied, this is an urgent indication for surgical exploration in the operating theatre.

In crush injury to the limbs, intravenous fluid replacement should be considered early. Muscle damage leads to rhabdomyolysis, myoglobinaemia, and hyperkalaemia (6).

Emergency department

Clinical examination of limb

After the primary survey, a repeat assessment of the limb should be performed. A photograph of the fracture wound should be added to the medical record if not already done. All hospitals are required to provide systems to enable upload of such photographs to the medical record in accordance with data protection regulations (4). Contaminants such as large foreign bodies are removed but irrigation is not performed. Antiseptics or antibiotics are not to be used in the wound dressing. Clean dressings should be reapplied if removed.

Compartment syndrome can occur in open fractures and clinicians should be aware of this possibility in the emergency department. A repeat assessment of the limb is independent of previous documented findings so that changes of arterial and neurological status can be identified promptly.

Following reassessment of the limb, temporary splints may be removed but, in many cases, a traction splint or vacuum splint may be the best way to support the limb pending definitive surgery.

Antibiotics

Although prompt administration of antibiotics after injury is essential, there is insufficient evidence to support prolonged administration (7). Antibiotics for 1 day appear as effective as 3–5 days (8–11).

A retrospective review of patients with Gustilo grade IIIB fractures showed that the majority of deep infections were caused by nosocomial organisms, most being resistant to the initial antibiotic prophylaxis aimed at environmental flora (11). This has led to our recommendation of a two-phase antibiotic protocol with a second wave of prophylaxis against nosocomial organisms at the time of definitive wound closure.

We recommend that trauma surgeons refer to local antibiotic guidelines, which should be written in conjunction with the microbiology department and pharmacy and take into account local epidemiology and formularies. Guidelines should include paediatric recommendations written with additional paediatric input. Doses for children are available in the paediatric British National Formulary (https://bnfc.nice.org.uk/).

We recommend local guidelines should be based on the following phased antibiotic regimen (only normal adult doses stated).

Phase 1

Within 1 hour of injury and continue until wound excision.

- First line:
  - (a) co-amoxiclav (1.2 g) 8-hourly intravenously (iv) **or**
  - (b) an intravenous cephalosporin, e.g. ceftriaxone 2 g daily.
- Patients with a history of non-severe penicillin allergy (e.g. rash) should receive a cephalosporin not co-amoxiclav.
- Those with a history of anaphylaxis or other severe reaction to penicillin should receive clindamycin 900 mg iv 8-hourly (+ gentamicin 3 mg/kg single dose for presumed Gustilo grade III fractures (12)).
- For patients at high risk of methicillin-resistant *Staphylococcus aureus* (MRSA) or those known to be positive for MRSA, a glycopeptide should be added, e.g. teicoplanin 800 mg iv daily (with extra loading dose after first 12 hours).
- Unusual environmental exposures should prompt early discussion with microbiology.

At the first excision of the wound, on induction of anaesthesia, a single dose of gentamicin 3 mg/kg[1] § should be added to the above (unless they have already received gentamicin in the past 16 hours).

---

[1] Gentamicin dosing is based on the patient's actual body weight. If the patient's actual weight is more than 20% above ideal body weight (IBW), the dosing weight (DW) can be determined as follows: DW = IBW + 0.4 × (actual weight − IBW). If underweight by more than 20% of IBW then DW = 0.4 × (IBW − actual weight).

IBW (kg) = (males 50 kg, females 45 kg) + 2.3 kg per inch over 5ft.

Further intra-operative doses of co-amoxiclav should be given if there is major blood loss (>10% blood volume) or if the procedure lasts more than 3 hours. Do not give additional doses of once-daily antibiotics, e.g. gentamicin, ceftriaxone, or teicoplanin, unless it has been more than 16 hours since the last dose).

Treatment with antibiotics after wound excision (phase 1) should continue for 24 hours.

Phase 2

♦ At the time of definitive skeletal stabilisation and definitive soft tissue coverage the patient should receive a single intravenous dose at induction of a glycopeptide, e.g. teicoplanin 800 mg (if it has been more than 12 hours since the last dose) plus gentamicin 3 mg/kg (if it has been more than 16 hours since the last dose). This is to provide cover for organisms selected out from initial prophylaxis and for nosocomial pathogens (13).

No further postoperative antibiotics are required.

Some authorities recommend 5 mg/kg gentamicin for prophylaxis (14). However, there is evidence that there may be an increased risk of nephrotoxicity when prophylactic gentamicin is introduced to protocols (15–17). A retrospective study of 167 open fractures showed that prophylactic gentamicin was not associated with acute kidney injury (AKI). AKI was associated with hypotension on admission and a higher Injury Severity Score (18). Potential nephrotoxicity should be balanced against the benefit of increasing the breadth and effectiveness of antimicrobial cover. Common practice in prophylaxis is to use a lower single dose of 3 mg/kg as suggested in this guideline.

Thromboprophylaxis

Venous thromboembolism (VTE) is a risk for any patient with major trauma or a lower limb injury. Surveillance studies indicate 58% of patients with major trauma are affected; advanced age and obesity add further to this risk (19). All patients must be considered for thromboprophylaxis. Pharmacological VTE prophylaxis is the most widely used method for trauma patients and is supported by national guidance, although caution is needed where patients are coagulopathic or there may be bleeding from associated vascular, intracranial, or visceral injuries (20). Low molecular weight heparins such as enoxaparin have been shown to be superior to low-dose heparin and are used for this purpose (21). New oral anticoagulants (NOACs) should be used with caution as the timing of definitive surgery may not be clear in the early stages of assessment and treatment. Mechanical devices such as intermittent calf pumps may not be appropriate on the injured limb as they may affect the damaged soft tissue envelope and are not applicable if external fixation is present. Similarly, foot impulse devices may not be appropriate if there is risk of increased bleeding from the wound. The most invasive mechanical prophylaxis against embolism is the inferior vena caval (IVC) filter, which is a device implanted in the inferior vena cava that prevents thrombi reaching the pulmonary vasculature. The clinical indications and period of retention for such devices are evolving and use is reserved currently for the high-risk patients who are not suitable for pharmacological methods of prophylaxis. In all cases, clinicians should refer to their local hospital guidelines and the NICE guidance on VTE (20).

Imaging of limb

Necessary imaging should be obtained without unnecessary delay. For isolated open fractures, orthogonal radiographs should include visualisation of the joint above and below the injured segment. Further cross-sectional imaging is valuable particularly in peri-articular injuries, e.g. tibial plateau fractures. In patients where an initial 'trauma CT' is indicated there should be protocols to maximise the useful information and minimise delay; the initial sequence should include a head to toes scanogram. This should be used with clinical correlation to direct further specific limb sequences during that initial CT examination.

CT angiography may be helpful if it can be performed while the patient is having the 'major trauma series' scan (4). Formal angiography may be useful in assessing vascular injury in preparation for free-flap reconstruction. However, angiography should not delay emergency revascularisation of an ischaemic limb; immediate surgical exploration and shunting is indicated if hard signs of vascular injury persist after any necessary restoration of limb alignment and joint reduction.

Transfer from the emergency department

The trauma team leader, in conjunction with relevant specialists, will determine the most appropriate destination for the patient. This will be either directly to the operating theatres, to the intensive care unit, or to the major trauma ward. This important decision must be made jointly between senior orthopaedic and senior plastic surgeons. However, in cases of multiple injuries, the presence of an open fracture should not preclude transfer to a specialist area of the hospital, e.g. the neurosciences unit, if other injuries take priority.

References

1. **National Clinical Guideline Centre (UK).** *Fractures (Complex): Assessment and Management.* London: National Institute for Health and Care Excellence (UK); 2016 Feb. NG37. https://www.nice.org.uk/guidance/ng37/chapter/Recommendations#hospital-settings

2. **ATLS Subcommittee, American College of Surgeons' Committee on Trauma and International ATLS working group.** Advanced Trauma Life Support (ATLS®): the ninth edition. J Trauma Acute Care Surg. 2013;74(5):1363–6.

3. **National Association of Emergency Medical Technicians US (NAEMT).** Musculoskeletal trauma, in: Prehospital Trauma Life Support. 8th ed. Burlington, MA: Jones and Bartlett Publishers, Inc; 2016.

4. **Gosselin RA, Roberts I, Gillespie WJ.** Antibiotics for preventing infection in open limb fractures. Cochrane Database of Systeatic Reviews. 2004; Issue 1, Art. No.: CD003764.

5. **Lack WD, Karunakar MA, Angerame MR, Seymour RB, Sims S, Kellam JF,** et al. Type III open tibia fractures: immediate antibiotic prophylaxis minimizes infection. J Orthop Trauma. 2015;29(1):1–6.

6. **Lee C, Porter K.** Prehospital management of lower limb fractures. Emergency Medicine Journal: EMJ. 2005;22(9):660–3.

7. **Hauser CJ, Adams CA, Jr,** Eachempati SR. Surgical Infection Society guideline: prophylactic antibiotic use in open fractures: an evidence-based guideline. Surg Infect (Larchmt). 2006;7(4):379–405.

8. **Chang Y, Kennedy SA, Bhandari M, Lopes LC, de Cassia Bergamaschi C, de Oliveira e Silva MC,** et al. Effects of antibiotic prophylaxis in patients with open fracture of the extremities: a systematic review of randomized controlled trials. JBJS Rev. 2015;3(6):pii:01874474-201503060-00002

9. **Isaac SM, Woods A, Danial IN, Mourkus H.** Antibiotic prophylaxis in adults with open tibial fractures: what is the evidence for duration of administration? A systematic review. J Foot Ankle Surg. 2016;55(1):146–50.

10. **Dellinger EP, Caplan ES, Weaver LD, Wertz MJ, Droppert BM, Hoyt N,** et al. Duration of preventive antibiotic administration for open extremity fractures. Arch Surg. 1988;123(3):333–9.

11. **Dunkel N, Pittet D, Tovmirzaeva L, Suva D, Bernard L, Lew D,** et al. Short duration of antibiotic prophylaxis in open fractures does not enhance risk of subsequent infection. Bone Joint J. 2013;95 B(6):831–7.

12. **Vasenius J, Tulikoura I, Vainionpaa S, Rokkanen P.** Clindamycin versus cloxacillin in the treatment of 240 open fractures. A randomized prospective study. Ann Chir Gynaecol. 1998;87(3):224–8.

13. **Glass GE, Barrett SP, Sanderson F, Pearse MF, Nanchahal J.** The microbiological basis for a revised antibiotic regimen in high-energy tibial fractures: preventing deep infections by nosocomial organisms. J Plast Reconstr Aesthet Surg. 2011;64(3):375–80.

14. **Bratzler DW, Dellinger EP, Olsen KM, Perl TM, Auwaerter PG, Bolon MK,** et al. Clinical practice guidelines for antimicrobial prophylaxis in surgery. Surgical Infections. 2013;14(1):73–156.

15. **Nielsen DV, Fedosova M, Hjortdal V, Jakobsen CJ.** Is single-dose prophylactic gentamicin associated with acute kidney injury in patients undergoing cardiac surgery? A matched-pair analysis. J Thorac Cardiovasc Surg. 2014;**148**(4):1634–9.

16. **Craxford S, Bayley E, Needoff M.** Antibiotic-associated complications following lower limb arthroplasty: a comparison of two prophylactic regimes. Eur J Orthop Surg Traumatol. 2014;**24**(4):539–43.

17. **Challagundla SR, Knox D, Hawkins A, Hamilton D, R Flynn, RWV,** et al. Renal impairment after high-dose flucloxacillin and single-dose gentamicin prophylaxis in patients undergoing elective hip and knee replacement. Nephrol Dial Transplant. 2013;**28**(3):612–19.

18. **Tessier JM, Moore B, Putty B, Gandhi RR, Duane TM.** Prophylactic gentamicin is not associated with acute kidney injury in patients with open fractures. Surg Infect (Larchmt). 2016;**17**(6):720–3.

19. **Geerts WH, Code KI, Jay RM, Chen E, Szalai JP.** A prospective study of venous thromboembolism after major trauma. N Engl J Med. 1994;**331**(24):1601–6.

20. **National Institute for Health and Care Excellence (NICE).** Venous thromboembolism: reducing the risk for patients in hospital. NICE Guideline NG89 (March 2018 updated August 2019). https://www.nice.org.uk/guidance/ng89/chapter/Recommendations

21. **Geerts WH, Jay RM, Code KI, Chen E, Szalai JP, Saibil EA,** et al. A comparison of low-dose heparin with low-molecular-weight heparin as prophylaxis against venous thromboembolism after major trauma. N Engl J Med. 1996;**335**(10):701–7.

Chapter 2

Timing of Wound Excision

Summary

1. Highly contaminated lower limb fractures should undergo immediate wound excision in theatre.
2. Wound excision should be performed jointly by consultant orthopaedic and plastic surgeons.
3. High-energy lower limb fractures (likely Gustilo–Anderson Type IIIA and IIIB), which are not highly contaminated, should undergo wound excision within 12 hours of injury and all other lower limb fractures should be excised within 24 hours of injury. The consultant orthoplastic surgical team are best placed to determine the timing for individual patients based on clinical assessment.

Introduction

The aim of wound excision is to remove contaminating debris and all devitalised tissue. This should reduce both the bacterial burden and available substrate for microbial colonisation, resulting in fewer deep surgical site infections. In turn, this will lead to improved patient outcomes. The timing of wound excision has been the subject of intense debate. In the past, guidelines have favoured wound excision within 6 hours based on historical animal and human studies. However, it is difficult to isolate the effect of timing alone owing to the many confounding factors, including patient characteristics, mechanism of injury, timing and type of antibiotics, and timing of soft tissue reconstruction.

Literature review

In 2016, the National Institute for Health and Care Excellence (NICE) performed a systematic review of the literature (1) with regard to timing of wound excision when managing open fractures. Two further reviews have followed (2, 3), both with methodological limitations. The NICE review identified no randomised controlled trials. Nine cohort studies were included, two prospective and seven retrospective. Thirty-one studies were excluded owing to inadequate adjustment for confounders and for not meeting the protocol criteria. A subsequent search identified a further retrospective study on timing of excision after 24 hours following injury (4).

The NICE review identified two studies suggesting no clinical difference in deep surgical site infection rates between early and late wound excision (6 or 8 hours or less versus more than 6 or 8 hours, respectively) (5, 6). Another study suggested low deep surgical site infection rate with early wound excision (less than 8 hours) (7). A further three studies suggested timing of wound excision is not a predictor of deep surgical site infection (8–10). In a large retrospective study of patients with open tibial fractures, primary wound excision beyond the first day of admission was associated with a significantly increased probability of amputation (11).

NICE have recommended that all open fractures should be excised jointly by consultant orthopaedic and plastic surgeons. A series comparing open fractures managed by a specialist centre versus those initially managed at local centres showed that the latter had increased complication rates and revision surgery (12). This is supported by another retrospective study, which found that patients with open ankles, initially treated at peripheral centres, undergo additional, potentially avoidable operations (13).

Using arbitrary time cut-offs rather than analysing time as a continuum reduces statistical power. Hull et al. looked retrospectively at the accumulative effect of delayed wound excision on deep surgical site infection rates (14). They reported a series of 364 consecutive patients with 459 open limb fractures. After controlling for confounding variables and considering all grades of fractures together, they found with each hour passing post-injury there was an increase in the odds ratio for infection of 1.033. When subdivided by fracture severity, a delay in the first wound excision had a greater effect on higher-grade fractures. Open fractures of the tibia had an increased odds ratio for infection of 2.44 compared with non-tibia sites and high-grade (IIIB and IIIC) had higher rates of infection than low-grade (II and IIIA) injuries. Therefore, high-grade fractures of the tibia where excision is delayed are at the greatest risk of developing deep infection. The NICE Guidance Development Group recommended that highly contaminated fractures such as those exposed to the aquatic environment or sustained in the agricultural environment should be excised immediately in theatre. High-grade open fractures (presumed grade IIIA or IIIB) should be excised within 12 hours and all other open fractures, excluding those of the hand, toes, and wrist, within 24 hours of the injury.

Economic considerations

No studies consider the economics or cost effectiveness of different timings. The NICE Guidance Development Group performed a cost analysis that explored the timing of initial wound excision with or without the presence of a plastic surgeon, timing of soft tissue cover, and provision of multiple theatre sessions. It found that as the delay to wound excision increased, so did the costs owing to increased complication rates. In addition, the increased staff costs to deliver early wound excision by consultant plastic surgeons alongside consultant orthopaedic surgeons are outweighed by the costs of potential complications if the patient is treated sequentially or inadequately.

Conclusion

The available evidence shows benefits of early wound excision. Timing of wound excision is largely modifiable unlike severity of injury and presence of gross contamination, which are both major risk factors. The NICE guidelines take account of the relative contributions of these risk factors and balance them with the potential risks of out-of-hours surgery alongside the health economic requirements of delivering a service.

References

1. **National Clinical Guideline Centre (UK).** Fractures (Complex): Assessment and Management. London: National Institute for Health and Care Excellence (UK); 2016 Feb. NG37. https://www.nice.org.uk/guidance/ng37/chapter/Recommendations#hospital-settings
2. **Prodromidis AD, Charalambous CP.** The 6-hour rule for surgical debridement of open tibial fractures: a systematic review and meta-analysis of infection and nonunion rates. J Orthop Trauma. 2016;**30**(7):397–402.
3. **Rozell JC, Connolly KP, Mehta S.** Timing of operative debridement in open fractures. Orthop Clin North Am. 2017;**48**(1):25–34.
4. **Duyos OA, Beaton-Comulada D, Davila-Parrilla A, Perez-Lopez JC, Ortiz K, Foy-Parrilla C,** et al. Management of open tibial shaft fractures: does the timing of surgery affect outcomes? J Am Acad Orthop Surg. 2017;**25**(3):230–8.
5. **Enninghorst N, McDougall D, Hunt JJ, Balogh ZJ.** Open tibia fractures: timely debridement leaves injury severity as the only determinant of poor outcome. The J Trauma. 2011;**70**(2):352–6.
6. **Harley BJ, Beaupre LA, Jones CA, Dulai SK, Weber DW.** The effect of time to definitive treatment on the rate of nonunion and infection in open fractures. J Orthop Trauma. 2002;**16**(7):484–90.
7. **Malhotra AK, Goldberg S, Graham J, Malhotra NR, Willis MC, Mounasamy V,** et al. Open extremity fractures: impact of delay in operative debridement and irrigation. J Trauma Acute Care Surg. 2014;**76**(5):1201–7.

8. Lack WD, Karunakar MA, Angerame MR, Seymour RB, Sims S, Kellam JF, et al. Type III open tibia fractures: immediate antibiotic prophylaxis minimizes infection. J Orthop Trauma. 2015;**29**(1):1–6.

9. Weber D, Dulai SK, Bergman J, Buckley R, Beaupre LA. Time to initial operative treatment following open fracture does not impact development of deep infection: a prospective cohort study of 736 subjects. J Orthop Trauma. 2014;**28**(11):613–9.

10. Charalambous CP, Siddique I, Zenios M, Roberts S, Samarji R, Paul A, et al. Early versus delayed surgical treatment of open tibial fractures: effect on the rates of infection and need of secondary surgical procedures to promote bone union. Injury. 2005;**36**(5):656–61.

11. Sears ED, Davis MM, Chung KC. Relationship between timing of emergency procedures and limb amputation in patients with open tibia fracture in the United States, 2003 to 2009. Plast Reconstr Surg. 2012;**130**(2):369–78.

12 Naique SB, Pearse M, Nanchahal J. Management of severe open tibial fractures: the need for combined orthopaedic and plastic surgical treatment in specialist centres. J Bone Joint Surg Br 2006;**88**(3):351–7.

13 Chummun S, Wright TC, Chapman TWL, Khan U. Outcome of the management of open ankle fractures in an ortho-plastic specialist centre. Injury Int. J. Care Injured 2015;**46**:1112–15.

14. Hull PD, Johnson SC, Stephen DJG, Kreder HJ, Jenkinson RJ. Delayed debridement of severe open fractures is associated with a higher rate of deep infection. Bone Joint J. 2014;**96**-B(3):379–84.

Chapter 3

Wound Excision

Summary

1. Assessment of tissue viability is difficult after open trauma and wound excision should be performed by consultant plastic and orthopaedic surgeons as a combined procedure.
2. Immediate surgical exploration is indicated in the presence of gross wound contamination, compartment syndrome, devascularised limb, or multiple injuries.
3. Wound extensions are used to facilitate wound excision and allow inspection of deeper structures. In the tibia these should follow fasciotomy lines.
4. Wound excision should be systematic to ensure all devitalised soft tissue and bone is removed whilst preserving the neurovascular bundles. Repeat wound excision may be required in the presence of tissues of doubtful viability whilst still respecting the timelines to reconstruction.
5. Low-pressure lavage with a high volume of tepid 0.9% saline completes the wound excision.
6. The injury is classified at the end of the final wound excision.
7. Closure of an open fracture wound should be a combined decision between orthopaedic and plastic consultants.
8. Definitive fracture fixation after wound excision should be undertaken as a distinctly separate operative procedure with re-prepping of the limb and opening of fixation instruments and implants at the time of stabilisation.

Introduction

Early, thorough wound excision of the traumatic wound is probably the most important step in the prevention of infection after an open limb fracture. Devitalised tissues and foreign material facilitate the growth of microorganisms and constitute a barrier for the host's defence mechanisms.

We made the decision that in this publication we would replace the term **debridement** with the term **wound excision**, both in our own narrative and when referring to the publications of others. This should lead the reader to the principle that successful separation of tissues that are contaminated or non-viable from those that are healthy and viable relies on surgical excision of the former. Surgical access to the area requiring excision will include an extension of the traumatic wound by incision. The change in terminology from **debridement** to **wound excision** then encourages the concept that completion of the process relies on more than just lavage and dilution of contaminants.

Surgical extension of the traumatic wound should be sufficient to allow a thorough assessment of all components of the injury and an accurate injury classification.

Limb preparation

Dressings applied in the emergency room should only be removed when the patient is in the operating theatre. The dressings and splint are removed, the zone of injury and limb perfusion are re-examined, and a 'social wash' or 'pre-wash' of the limb is performed with a soapy chlorhexidine solution prior to formal prepping. A Cochrane review of preoperative bathing or showering with antiseptics in clean surgery provided no clear evidence of a reduction in surgical site infections (1). However, the surface of the injured limb is frequently contaminated with particulate matter and dried blood, and a gentle pre-wash creates a clean surface ready for formal skin antisepsis. The social wash also serves to identify any other injuries to the limb that may not have been readily apparent at initial assessment. The pre-wash is ideally performed in the anaesthetic room after induction to maintain theatre cleanliness. A tourniquet may be applied the limb and inflated for selected parts of the procedure. Photographs of open fracture wounds should be taken after the social wash, before the open wound is excised and at other key stages of management such as the end of wound excision. The photographs should be stored as part of the patient's record (2, 3).

The patient is then transferred to the operating table and skin antisepsis undertaken to reduce the presence of microorganisms. Alcohol-based preparations have been found to be more effective for other surgical procedures (4). When alcoholic solutions are used, care must be taken to avoid contact with the open wound and pooling beneath a tourniquet.

The surgical equipment used for performing the wound excision must be kept separate from the equipment for the subsequent fracture stabilisation to facilitate the conversion of the contaminated wound into a clean wound and to reduce the risk of contaminating the fracture hardware. If primary wound closure or definitive soft tissue cover and definitive fracture fixation is anticipated at the end of the wound excision, the limb should be formally re-prepped and draped for the second stage with new sterile equipment.

Wound extension

Elastic recoil of the tissues at the moment of injury and first aid measures to re-align and splint the limb may result in contaminated tissues remaining within the wound and the extent of tissue damage and contamination will not be immediately obvious. Formal wound extension is usually required to allow a systematic examination of the tissues and exposure of the fracture fragments. Regardless of the location of the traumatic wound, wound extensions must follow the fasciotomy lines (Figure 3.1). The majority of open tibial wounds are

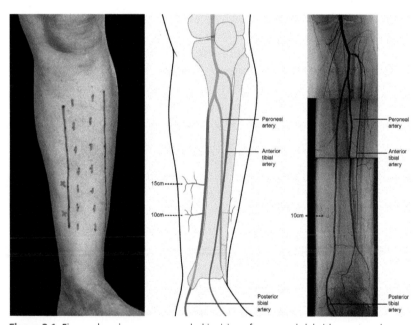

Figure 3.1 Figure showing recommended incisions for wound debridement and fasciotomies in the leg. The medial incision alone is usually sufficient for wound excision and preserves the perforators arising from the posterior tibial vessels, which form the basis of local fasciocutanoeus flaps. It also provides access to the posterior tibial artery and venae commitans when required as recipient vessels for free flaps. The lateral incision is used for decompression of the anterior and peroneal compartments in patients with compartment syndrome. (A) Margins of subcutaneous border of the tibia marked in green, access incisions marked in blue, and perforators arising from the medial side as red crosses. (B) Line drawing depicting the location of the perforators, with approximate indicative distances from the tip of the medial malleolus. (C) Montage of arteriogram.

located in the anteromedial aspect of the tibia, with varying degrees of exposure of the tibial bone. The medial fasciotomy extension avoids further inadvertent exposure of the tibia and protects the posterior tibial artery perforators, which are vital for a local fasciocutaneous flap. The medial extension also allows inspection of the posterior tibial vessels and nerve if required and provides ready access to the recipient vessels for free flaps. It is important that the wound extensions are performed in the subfascial plane to avoid degloving.

Tissue excision

Assessment of tissue viability is difficult and wound excision should be performed jointly by consultant plastic and orthopaedic surgeons (2). A systematic approach to wound excision is recommended, working from the wound margin to the centre and from the superficial structures to the deep layers of the wound. The wound extensions must allow inspection of the deep posterior muscle compartment in severe injuries to identify devitalised muscle, foreign material, and bone fragments driven into the tissues at the time of injury. A gradient of tissue damage is usually encountered, with obvious non-viable tissue at the points of greatest injury, surrounded by zones of variable tissue damage.

Tourniquet use is determined by surgical preference. A bloodless field allows identification of major neurovascular structures, facilitates soft tissue wound excision by avoiding blood staining, and also limits blood loss. However, prolonged tourniquet times should be avoided to prevent ischaemia and reperfusion injury (5). The tourniquet must be deflated after wound excision to formally assess tissue viability and achieve haemostasis.

Skin is relatively resilient but is vulnerable to direct crush and torsion/avulsion injuries, which may damage the septocutaneous and musculocutaneous perforators and cause necrosis. Early signs of skin necrosis include fixed staining (non-blanching on digital pressure) or subcutaneous vein thrombosis, but the extent of necrosis may be difficult to determine within the first 24–48 hours of injury. Contused skin at the margins of the open wound should be carefully excised to leave edges that bleed from the dermis.

Subcutaneous fat injury is easily missed, with potentially serious consequences. Fat is vulnerable to injury by direct compression and the extent of fat necrosis will often extend beyond the skin injury (see Chapter 4).

Devitalised muscle can be difficult to assess and the traditional method of assessment of is by the four 'C's: colour (pink not blue), contraction, consistency (devitalised muscle tears in the forceps during retraction), and capacity to bleed. A 1956 study of excised specimens from 12 war wounds found that consistency, contractility, and capacity to bleed were reliable predictors of muscle damage, whilst the colour was not (6). However, a more recent histopathological study showed that neither the four Cs nor the surgeons' impression correlated with histologic appearance (7). The analysis of 36 muscle biopsies found that 60% of specimens labelled borderline or necrotic by the surgeon were shown to comprise normal muscle on histopathological examination (7). These findings undermine current wound excision practices and suggest that surgeons may excise potentially viable muscle. Equally, retained dead muscle may lead to deep infection, emphasising the importance of consultant surgeons experienced in trauma management working together to achieve optimal outcomes.

Cortical bone has a relatively poor blood supply and assessment of viability is difficult. Small bone fragments with tenuous soft tissue attachments, which dislodge or separate easily during a steady pull (the 'tug test'), should be removed owing to their poor blood supply. Larger bone fragments should be carefully inspected for fracture edge or cortical bleeding. Fracture fragments should not be regarded as bone graft. Necrotic fragments and avascular fracture ends are unlikely to contribute to fracture union and may serve only as a nidus for infection. If there is doubt regarding the viability of bone ends or fragments, they should probably be removed. Large articular cartilage fragments attached to cancellous bone may be preserved, provided they are large enough to contribute to articular stability. Such fragments should be thoroughly cleaned with scrubbing, curettage, and lavage prior to reduction and fixation with absolute stability.

The main bone ends should be carefully delivered through the wound or appropriate wound extensions and the extent of periosteal stripping determined. The bone ends are cleared of haematoma with curettes and saline irrigation, and the medullary canal is inspected for debris. Occasionally road debris is embedded in the bone ends and must be meticulously removed. Fracture viability is inferred from the capacity of the bone ends to bleed, which is seen as a punctate ooze. Care must be taken not to mistake bleeding from the medullary canal for viability from a stripped fracture end, and periodic saline irrigation and suction help maintain visibility. Non-viable fracture ends may require resection with a cooled saw blade or large rongeur until bleeding bone is seen.

Wound irrigation

The aims of irrigation are to remove blood and particulate debris, to reduce the bacterial count, and facilitate tissue visibility. However, irrigation of open wounds has the potential to drive debris and bacteria into the deep layers of the wound (8) and should only be undertaken after adequate surgical removal of macroscopic contaminants and devitalised tissue. The FLOW study examined the effect of irrigation pressures and the use of soap or saline solutions in open fracture wounds (9). The authors found no benefit with high-pressure lavage and noted increased re-operation rates with soap solution. We recommend the use of a minimum of 3 litres of low-pressure saline lavage aided with digital agitation of the tissues as appropriate.

Wound cultures

Wound cultures from wound excision of acute open fractures do not directly correlate with later infection. One study of cultures taken during the initial wound excision highlighted either no growth (76%) or skin flora only (26%), and no isolates were implicated with cases of subsequent infection (10). In another study of 245 cases of open fracture, post-wound excision cultures were shown to have a greater prognostic value than that of pre-wound excision culture (11). However, of the cases that became infected, the infecting organism was present on post-wound excision cultures only 42% of the time. The author concluded that pre-wound excision and post-wound excision bacterial cultures from open fracture wounds are of essentially no value (11).

Classification of open fractures

Classifying open fractures is an important step in assessing the severity of the injury, directing treatment and determining prognosis. The development of an all-encompassing classification system for open fractures has proven difficult due to the difficulties of accurately characterising the multiple tissues involved in the injury. Although several classification systems for open fractures have been proposed, the Gustilo–Anderson classification first described in 1976 for open tibial fractures is the most widely used (12). After reviewing their initial classification of the most severe open injuries, Gustilo et al. subsequently modified the classification system into its current form in 1984 and the grading has since been applied to open fractures in all regions of the body (13, 14).

Type I fractures are low-energy injuries with a wound of less than 1 cm and no muscle damage or contamination. Typical fracture patterns include spiral and oblique fractures with minimal comminution.

Type II fractures are higher-energy injuries with a wound greater than 1 cm, mild-to-moderate muscle trauma, periosteal stripping, and contamination. The fracture patterns reflect the higher energy and include bending wedge, segmental, and comminuted fractures.

Type III injuries reflect high-energy trauma and the original classification was modified into three subtypes in order of worsening prognosis (13).

Type IIIA are due to high-energy trauma, irrespective of the size of the wound but there is adequate soft tissue coverage of the fractured bone despite extensive soft tissue laceration or flaps.

Type IIIB fractures are associated with more extensive soft tissue injury loss, periosteal stripping, and bone exposure necessitating formal soft tissue cover. This is usually associated with massive contamination.

Type IIIC injuries are open fractures associated with arterial injury requiring repair, i.e. a devascularised limb.

Although the Gustilo–Anderson classification has prognostic value for predicting infection (14), the grading is not ideal and has been shown to have relatively poor inter-observer reliability (15). In addition, there are only two categories of severe fractures (types IIIB and IIIC), which cannot be subclassified based on potentially important injury characteristics (16). In view of the limitations of the Gustilo–Anderson classification, assessment of all open fractures should include the mechanism of injury, the appearance of the soft tissue envelope and its condition in the operating room, the level of likely bacterial contamination, and the specific characteristics of the fracture (14). Hence the definitive assessment of an open fracture is best accomplished after formal surgical exploration and wound excision rather than in the emergency department (17).

Wound closure

Traditionally, delayed wound closure was the accepted approach to prevent deep infection in open fractures, particularly infection caused by *Clostridia* species or other anaerobic organisms (18). Primary wound closure in selected cases has the potential advantage of protection against hospital-acquired (nosocomial) infections. In addition, immediate wound closure may reduce the number of surgeries required and allow earlier mobilisation and discharge from hospital (19). A number of studies have suggested that primary closure in appropriately selected subjects results in acceptable patient outcomes with low rates of infection (19, 20). The difficulty lies in defining which wounds are amenable to early closure. Immediate wound closure should only be performed after a joint decision by experienced orthopaedic and plastic consultants working at a high-volume trauma centre, and patients must be closely monitored to assess for surgical site infection.

References

1. **Webster and S. Osbourne.** Preoperative bathing or showering with skin antiseptics to prevent surgical site infection. Cochrane Database of Systematic Reviews, 2015. DOI:10.1002/14651858.CD004985.pub5

2. **National Clinical Guideline Centre (UK).** *Fractures (Complex): Assessment and Management.* London: National Institute for Health and Care Excellence (UK); 2016 Feb. NG37. https://www.nice.org.uk/guidance/ng37/chapter/Recommendations#hospital-settings

3. **British Orthopaedic Association.** BOAST—Open fractures. London: BOA; December 2017. https://www.boa.ac.uk/resources/boast-4-pdf.html

4. **Dumville JC, McFarlane E, Edwards P, Lipp A, Holmes A,** Preoperative skin antiseptics for preventing surgical wound infections after clean surgery. Cochrane Database Syst Rev. 2015(4):Cd003949.

5. **Noordin S, McEwen JA, Kragh JF Jr, Eisen A, Masri BA.** Surgical tourniquets in orthopaedics. J Bone Joint Surg Am. 2009;**91**(12):2958–67.

6. **Artz CP, Sako Y and Scully RE.** An evaluation of the surgeon's criteria for determining the viability of muscle during debridement. AMA Arch Surg. 1956;**73**(6):1031–5.

7. **Sassoon A, Riehl J, Rich A, Langford J, Haidukewych G, Pearl G, Koval KJ.** Muscle viability revisited: are we removing normal muscle? A critical evaluation of dogmatic debridement. J Orthop Trauma. 2016;**30**(1):17–21.

8. **Hassinger, SM, Harding G, Wongworawat MD.** High-pressure pulsatile lavage propagates bacteria into soft tissue. Clin Orthop Relat Res. 2005;**439**:27–31.

9. **FLOW Investigators, Bhandari M, Jeray KJ, Petrisor BA, Devereaux PJ, Heels-Ansdell D., et al.,** A trial of wound irrigation in the initial management of open fracture wounds. N Engl J Med. 2015;**373**(27):2629–41.

10. **Valenziano CP, Chattar-Cora D, O'Neill A, Hubli EH, Cudjoe EA.** Efficacy of primary wound cultures in long bone open extremity fractures: are they of any value? Arch Orthop Trauma Surg. 2002;**122**(5):259–61.

11. **Lee, J.** Efficacy of cultures in the management of open fractures. Clin Orthop Relat Res. 1997(339):71–5.

12. **Gustilo RB, Anderson JT.** Prevention of infection in the treatment of one thousand and twenty-five open fractures of long bones: retrospective and prospective analyses. J Bone Joint Surg Am. 1976;**58**(4):453–8.

13. **Gustilo RB, Mendoza RM, Williams DN.** Problems in the management of type III (severe) open fractures: a new classification of type III open fractures. J Trauma. 1984;**24**(8):742–6.

14. **Kim PH, Leopold SS.** In brief: Gustilo-Anderson classification. [corrected]. Clin Orthop Relat Res. 2012;**470**(11):3270–4.

15. **Brumback RJ, Jones AL.** Interobserver agreement in the classification of open fractures of the tibia. The results of a survey of two hundred and forty-five orthopaedic surgeons. J Bone Joint Surg Am. 1994;**76**(8):1162–6.

16. **Agel J, Evans AR, Marsh JL, Decoster TA, Lundy DW, Kellam JF, et al.,** The OTA open fracture classification: a study of reliability and agreement. Journal of Orthopaedic Trauma. 2013;**27**(7):379–84.

17. **Okike K, Bhattacharyya T.** Trends in the management of open fractures. A critical analysis. J Bone Joint Surg Am. 2006;**88**(12):2739–48.

18. **Hampton OP Jr.** Basic principles in management of open fractures. J Am Med Assoc. 1955;**159**(5):417–19.

19. **Scharfenberger AV, Alabassi K, Smith S, Weber D, Dulai SK, Bergman JW,** et al. Primary wound closure after open fracture: a prospective cohort study examining nonunion and deep infection. JOrthop Trauma. 2017;**31**(3):121–6.

20. **Jenkinson RJ, Kiss A, Johnson S, Stephen DJ, Kreder HJ.** Delayed wound closure increases deep-infection rate associated with lower-grade open fractures: a propensity-matched cohort study. J Bone Joint Surg Am. 2014;**96**(5):380–6.

Chapter 4

Degloving Injuries

Summary

1. Degloving of the limb occurs in the plane superficial to the deep fascia and the extent of injury is often underestimated.

2. Thrombosis of the subcutaneous veins usually indicates the need to excise the overlying skin.

3. Circumferentially degloved skin is not viable.

4. In severe injuries, multiplanar degloving can occur with variable involvement of individual muscles, which may be stripped from the bone. Under these circumstances, a second look is usually necessary.

5. It may be appropriate to offer patients with severe multiplanar degloving over a wide zone primary amputation within 72 hours of the injury.

6. Large collections (greater than 50 ml) associated with Morel–Lavallée lesions may be best treated by surgical evacuation rather than aspiration.

Introduction

Degloving is often associated with high-energy injuries. It occurs when the skin surface is subjected to forces, including torsion, crush, avulsion, or a combination of these. The soft tissues are sheared along single or multiple tissue planes, depending on the severity of the injury. In uniplanar injuries, degloving occurs between the subcutaneous fat and deep fascia. By contrast, in multiplanar injuries tissues are disrupted between and within muscle groups and between muscle and bone. Therefore, multiplanar degloving injuries represent a much more severe group. Both trans-muscular and intermuscular perforating vessels that normally perfuse the skin are avulsed during the degloving process, resulting in necrosis of the overlying skin. Necrosis of the degloved tissues may evolve over time and, whilst the underlying mechanisms remain largely unknown, venous congestion and inflammatory cell infiltrate may contribute and subjacent haematoma leads to production of proinflammatory cytokines and free radicals (1). Whilst evacuation of any haematoma may help salvage threatened skin, the mainstay of treatment remains excision of non-viable tissues and subsequent reconstruction.

Patterns of injury

The viability of the degloved tissues can be difficult to assess, and grading systems based on the degree of injury to the subcutaneous veins have been devised to help decide how best to salvage the affected tissues (2, 3). Intra- and subdermal thrombosis manifests as 'fixed staining'. This refers to the state of the skin on clinical inspection where there is a spectrum of discolouration of the skin. The colour can vary from red to blue but fails to blanch on digital pressure. Intravenous fluorescein may delineate non-viable tissues more accurately (4) but requires specialised equipment, carries a small risk of anaphylaxis, and has poor specificity.

In the clinical setting, the most useful classification system describes four patterns of degloving (3):

1. localised degloving;
2. non-circumferential, single plane degloving;
3. single plane, circumferential degloving;
4. circumferential and multiplanar degloving.

Over bony prominences, such as malleoli and condyles, pattern 1 can be associated with soft tissue loss because the mechanism of injury that usually causes degloving in these areas can result in tissue abrasion and avulsion. Whilst patterns 2, 3, and 4 can present as closed injuries, in practice, pattern 4 usually presents as an open wound. Circumferentially degloved skin is usually not viable as it will have been stripped of the perforators upon which it survives. Multiple patterns may co-exist in some patients and multiplanar injuries can occur in the absence of circumferential degloving. Patients with a wide zone of multiplanar degloving associated with a segmental tibial fracture may be best served by a primary amputation. Under some circumstances it may be appropriate to use free tissue transfer to achieve soft tissue coverage of the residual limb to enable a trans-tibial rather than through-knee amputation or to consider using spare parts from the distal part of the limb (5).

Management

Degloving injuries require definitive reconstructive surgery, which comprises excision of devitalised tissue and application of meshed split thickness skin graft, with flap coverage for exposed bone and fractures. The devitalised skin should be assessed clinically (as previously described) and carefully marked with a pen. The area is then excised systematically as per the approach used for wound excision (see Chapter 3). The soft tissues are assessed from superficial to deep in turn. On occasions when the soft tissue damage is difficult to assess, a second look should be undertaken 24–48 hours later when the devitalised tissues will have declared themselves. However, a general principle in open fracture management is that open fractures should be covered as soon as possible, and certainly within 72 hours. Therefore, repeated wound excisions are best avoided if possible (6).

At the end of soft tissue wound excision, conditions should be akin to those encountered during elective surgical wounds and meshed split thickness skin graft can be applied if appropriate. Skin grafting should not be performed if there is an underlying exposed fracture, which should instead be covered with a flap. Occasionally, the degloved skin can be used as a source of skin graft if it has not been traumatised directly. Some authors have reported the use of meshed split thickness autograft supplemented with overlying allograft or with an underlying dermal substitute such as Integra˚ (7). Full thickness skin grafting has also been described (8, 9). However, there is limited evidence to support these techniques and outcomes are likely unreliable.

We recommend the use of negative pressure wound therapy (NPWT) to secure the skin grafts (10). This offers the benefits of securing the graft to the recipient wound bed, which is often irregular, thus reducing the risk of fluid collections under the graft and maximising graft take (11, 12). A comparative study has shown that negative pressure treatment led to reduced requirement for repeated skin grafts and improved overall graft survival (12). A subsequent clinical trial found that NPWT also improved the qualitative appearance of split thickness skin grafts compared with standard dressings (13).

Closed degloving can present as post-traumatic subcutaneous fluid collections and diagnosis may be delayed several days to months following injury. Delayed diagnosis and treatment often results in full thickness necrosis due to compromised vascular supply of the avulsed skin flap. A specific type of closed degloving injury, where the subdermal fat is sheared from its underlying fascia and is associated with an effusion containing haematoma, lymphatic fluid, and necrotic fat, is known as the Morel–Lavallée lesion (14). These tend to occur in polytrauma patients and are associated with a high rate of infection, especially if there is an underlying fracture (15). Early diagnosis (by MRI) and treatment of closed degloving injuries are important to prevent infection, extensive skin necrosis, and chronic recurrence (16). Management options include aspiration and insertion of vacuum drains, or wound excision with or without sclerosing agents, followed by external compression. A retrospective study of 87 Morel–Lavallée lesions found that percutaneous aspiration had higher rates of recurrence (56%) compared with the observation and operative groups (19% and 15%, respectively) (17). Furthermore, based on their observation that aspiration of more than 50 ml of fluid is associated with a higher rate of recurrence (83% vs 33%), the authors recommended that lesions containing more than 50 ml should be managed surgically.

Conclusion

The standard of care for the treatment of degloved soft tissues remains excision of the devitalised tissues and reconstruction. The margin of excision can be difficult to determine. Fixed staining and thrombosis of the subcutaneous veins are indicative of skin that will not survive. Circumferentially degloved skin does not survive and the patient with multiplanar degloving should undergo meticulous and systematic excision of all the non-viable muscle and skin. A second look procedure may be necessary 24–48 hours later. Whilst large defects may be successfully reconstructed with free tissue transfer, it may be appropriate to offer patients with severe injuries a primary amputation.

References

1. **Glass GE, Nanchahal J.** Why haematomas cause flap failure: an evidence-based paradigm. J Plast Reconstr Aesthet Surg. 2012;**65**(7):903–10.
2. **Waikakul S.** Revascularization of degloving injuries of the limbs. Injury. 1997;**28**(4):271–4.
3. **Arnez ZM, Khan U, Tyler MP.** Classification of soft-tissue degloving in limb trauma. J Plast Reconstr Aesthet Surg. 2010;**63**(11):1865–9.
4. **Lim H, Han DH, Lee IJ, Park MC.** A simple strategy in avulsion flap injury: prediction of flap viability using Wood's lamp illumination and resurfacing with a full-thickness skin graft. Arch Plast Surg. 2014;**41**(2):126–32.
5. **Ghali S, Harris PA, Khan U, Pearse M, Nanchahal J.** Leg length preservation with pedicled fillet of foot flaps after traumatic amputations. Plast Reconstr Surg. 2005;**115**(2):498–505.
6. **Park SH, Silva M, Bahk WJ, McKellop H, Lieberman JR.** Effect of repeated irrigation and debridement on fracture healing in an animal model. J Orthop Res. 2002;**20**(6):1197–204.
7. **Violas P, Abid A, Darodes P, Galinier P, de Gauzy JS, Cahuzac JP.** Integra artificial skin in the management of severe tissue defects, including bone exposure, in injured children. J Pediatr Orthop B. 2005;**14**(5):381–4.
8. **Yan H, Gao W, Li Z, Wang C, Liu S, Zhang F,** et al. The management of degloving injury of lower extremities: technical refinement and classification. J Trauma Acute Care Surg. 2013;**74**(2):604–10.
9. **Sakai G, Suzuki T, Hishikawa T, Shirai Y, Kurozumi T, Shindo M.** Primary reattachment of avulsed skin flaps with negative pressure wound therapy in degloving injuries of the lower extremity. Injury. 2017;**48**(1):137–41.

10. **Azzopardi EA, Boyce DE, Dickson WA, Azzopardi E, Laing JH, Whitaker IS**, et al. Application of topical negative pressure (vacuum-assisted closure) to split-thickness skin grafts: a structured evidence-based review. Ann Plast Surg. 2013;70(1):23–9.

11. **Bovill E, Banwell PE, Teot L, Eriksson E, Song C, Mahoney J**, et al. Topical negative pressure wound therapy: a review of its role and guidelines for its use in the management of acute wounds. Int Wound J. 2008;5(4):511–29.

12. **Scherer LA, Shiver S, Chang M, Meredith JW, Owings JT.** The vacuum assisted closure device: a method of securing skin grafts and improving graft survival. Arch Surg. 2002;137(8):930–3; discussion 933–4.

13. **Moisidis E, Heath T, Boorer C, Ho K, Deva AK.** A prospective, blinded, randomized, controlled clinical trial of topical negative pressure use in skin grafting. Plast Reconstr Surg. 2004;114(4):917–22.

14. **Bonilla-Yoon I, Masih S, Patel DB, White EA, Levine BD, Chow K**, et al. The Morel-Lavallee lesion: pathophysiology, clinical presentation, imaging features, and treatment options. Emerg Radiol. 2014;21(1):35–43.

15. **Lekuya HM, Alenyo R, Kajja I, Bangirana A, Mbiine R, Deng AN**, et al. Degloving injuries with versus without underlying fracture in a sub-Saharan African tertiary hospital: a prospective observational study. J Orthop Surg Res. 2018;13(1):2.

16. **Scolaro JA, Chao T, Zamorano DP.** The Morel-Lavallée lesion: diagnosis and management. J Am Acad Orthop Surg. 2016;24(10):667–72.

17. **Nickerson TP, Zielinski MD, Jenkins DH, Schiller HJ.** The Mayo Clinic experience with Morel-Lavallée lesions: establishment of a practice management guideline. J Trauma Acute Care Surg. 2014;76(2):493–7.

Chapter 5

Temporary Wound Dressings

Summary

1. Consider a saline-soaked dressing covered with an occlusive layer for open fractures in prehospital settings and in the emergency department.
2. Following initial wound excision, if the wound cannot be closed primarily, use a simple non-adherent dressing.
3. When internal fixation is used, perform definitive soft tissue cover at the same time.
4. Prolonged application of negative pressure wound therapy (NPWT) should not be used to downgrade the requirements for definitive soft tissue reconstruction, which should be performed within 72 hours of injury.

Introduction

Temporary dressings are used to cover the wound from the time of injury through to definitive soft tissue closure. Frequent dressing changes should be avoided to reduce contamination by nosocomial organisms.

Immediately after injury, the wound is contaminated by organisms from the environment at the time of the trauma. However, the available evidence suggests that environmental contamination does not reflect the organisms typically responsible for subsequent deep tissue infection (1), except in specific areas such as farmyard and aquatic conditions. Therefore, the initial dressing should be simple to apply and maintain tissue viability by preventing desiccation, e.g. gauze soaked in normal saline and covered with an occlusive film as per the National Institute for Health and Care Excellence (NICE) guidance (2). Following wound excision, if immediate soft tissue cover cannot be achieved, a simple non-adherent dressing should be applied. NICE previously recommended the application of negative pressure wound therapy (NPWT) (2).

NPWT

Popularised by the first English language publications in the late 1980s and 1990s (3–5) NPWT is a closed system that applies suction to a deformable filler material in contact with a wound bed, producing positive pressure with micro-scopic focal areas of negative pressure where partially deformed filler pores abut the wound (6,7). NPWT works by a combination of macromechanical deformation, micromechanical deformation (stimulating mesenchymal mechanoreceptor-mediated proliferation and differentiation), permissive hypoxia-mediated angiogenesis (as a consequence of positive pressure to the wound bed), and the removal of oedema (8). At a molecular level NPWT sup-presses the expression of pro-inflammatory cytokines TNF and IL-1β and pro-motes expression of anti-inflammatory cytokines such as IL-10 and growth factors VEGF and TGF-β (9).

Therapy variables include the magnitude of negative pressure, the periodicity of application of negative pressure (continuous or intermittent), the material and deformational properties of the wound filler, and the use of an additional interface layer between the wound filler and wound bed, which may reduce granulation tissue ingrowth into the filler, confer antibacterial properties, and influence the deformational characteristics of the wound filler and the trans-mission of pressure to the wound bed (10). Whilst early studies reported en-hanced local blood flow with the use of an intermittent NPWT regimen (the 5 minutes on; 2 minutes off regime), the conclusions drawn from these data have been contested (5). Furthermore, whilst there is some evidence to suggest that intermittent application of NPWT may enhance wound healing in experi-mental models, this has not yet translated into a reliable therapeutic strategy (11,12). The available evidence for the influence of magnitude of negative pres-sure would suggest that –80 mmHg should be used as a default (13) as higher pressures are unlikely to confer additional clinical advantage and may even be detrimental to local tissue perfusion (14). The most commonly utilised wound filler is polyurethane (PU) foam. Under topical negative pressure the collaps-ible porous structure results in macromechanical wound deformation that may not be desirable in some areas, for example, a flexure crease over a joint. Additionally the porosity encourages granulation tissue ingrowth that leads to painful dressing changes as friable, bleeding tissue within the porous struc-ture is pulled from the wound as the dressing is changed. The limited ability of PU foam to conform to complex wound geometry has led to the use of gauze, such as polyhexanide-impregnated Kerlix™ as an alternative filler (15) without demonstrable differences in macro- and micromechanical wound deformation and pressure transduction (16, 17). Whilst the use of a single layer of inter-face material probably makes little difference to the application of pressure to the wound bed, non-adherent interface materials may be used to protect vital structures such as vessels and nerves.

The influence of NPWT on the bacteriology of the subjacent wound remains controversial. Experimentally, acute, chronic, and pre-contaminated wounds have all been investigated to answer this question, but intermittent surgical wound excision and the simultaneous use of systemic antibiotics have complicated data analysis and interpretation. Early studies hypothesised that NPWT suppressed bacterial growth, although more recent data suggest that this is an oversimplification. A recent systematic review aimed at establishing whether NPWT acts in part by improving bacterial clearance of the wound included 20 studies of which 10 were experimental studies, 4 were randomised controlled trials, and 6 clinical series.

Four additional studies (2 experimental studies and 2 clinical series) evaluated NPWT when used with periodic installation of antibacterial solutions. The authors concluded that the influence of NPWT on bacterial growth kinetics is probably species-specific. NPWT may selectively suppress the replication of Gram negative rods such as *Pseudomonas* spp. thereby depopulating the niche that is then filled by Gram positive cocci (18). The solution to this problem may lie in the use of antibacterial wound fillers and interface materials such as silver-impregnated foam and gauze. Whilst one study reported that the use of a silver-impregnated interface markedly suppressed growth of *Staphylococcus aureus* (19), corroborative data are, as yet, lacking.

NPWT works as a closed system. Leaks in the transparent membrane result in the continuous inflow of air from the external environment, risking contamination and wound desiccation. The NPWT pump sounds an alarm when the seal is breached. Maintenance of the seal can be challenging where the wound geometry is complex or where adjacent orifices preclude a reliable seal. Wounds under continuous (or intermittent) suction risk large losses of fluid, including blood. Therefore, it is important to examine the contents of the reservoir and document volumes collected at regular intervals and to take the patient back to the operating theatre should any concerns be raised over ongoing losses.

What is the evidence for NPWT in open fractures?

Several series have evaluated the use of NPWT in the immediate management of open fractures, i.e. the use of NPWT after the first surgical wound excision in those wounds that cannot be closed by direct suturing of the wound edges. The outcomes included infection, the subsequent reconstructive requirement of the wound, and the permissible delay between injury and definitive reconstruction.

NPWT and deep tissue infection

A prospective study of 58 patients with 62 open fractures randomised to NPWT or control (standard dressings) with wound excision and dressing changes every 48–72 hours until definitive closure reported 2 deep infections among 37 patients in the NPWT cohort and 7 deep infections among 25 patients in the control cohort. Overall, NPWT resulted in a significant reduction in deep infections, with an odds ratio of 0.199 (20). A retrospective cohort study of 229 open tibial fractures concluded that, when compared with conventional dressings, the use of NPWT reduced the rate of deep tissue infection by 80% (21). However, a UK-based, multicentre randomised controlled trial compared NPWT with standard dressings in 460 participants with lower limb open fractures of Gustilo–Anderson grade II (15%) or III (85%). Approximately 82% of the participants had tibial fractures. The investigators found no difference in self-reported disability rating index (DRI 45.5 NPWT, 42.4 standard dressing) or deep surgical site infection rates (7.1% NPWT, 8.1% standard dressing) at 12 months following injury, with superficial surgical site infections rates within 3 months of injury also being similar between the two groups (15.5 NPWT, 14.1% standard dressings) (22). The authors found that NPWT was not cost effective in improving outcomes.

NPWT and the subsequent reconstructive requirement of the wound

There is little evidence that the use of NPWT downgrades the reconstructive requirements of the wound. A prospective study of 16 patients with high-energy open fractures concluded that the use of NPWT is a useful temporising adjunct and does not downgrade the reconstructive requirements (23). Retrospective studies have reported that NPWT can be used to promote granulation tissue through prolonged application and thereby reduce the requirement for flap coverage (24–27), but most report unacceptably high deep infection rates.

NPWT and the permissible delay to definitive reconstruction

A retrospective study of 103 patients and 105 free tissue transfers for (mainly Gustilo–Anderson IIIB and IIIC) open lower limb fractures concluded that NPWT did not permit a delay in definitive soft tissue reconstruction as increased rates of flap take-back, failure, and deep metalwork infection were noted in the NPWT cohort after 72 hours (28). Whilst smaller retrospective series have reached various conclusions regarding permissible delay (29–31), the weight of evidence analysed and presented in the NICE Guideline concluded that definitive reconstruction should be undertaken within 72 hours (2).

Incisional NPWT over open fractures closed directly

A study of 249 patients with 263 lower extremity fractures (pilon, tibial plateau, and calcaneal) considered to be at high risk for wound dehiscence following definitive open reduction and internal fixation reported that the use of prophylactic NPWT over the closed incision significantly reduced wound dehiscence and risk of subsequent infection (32). However, a multicentre randomised controlled trial with 1548 participants found no difference in the deep surgical site infection rates at 30 and 90 days, patient-reported disability, health-related quality of life, surgical scar assessment, or chronic pain (33, 34). At 30 days, deep surgical site infection occurred in 5.84% of patients treated with NPWT compared with 6.68% of patients in the standard dressing group; absolute risk difference, −0.77%[95%CI, −3.19% to 1.66%]; $P = .52$) (34).

Other dressing modalities

A small uncontrolled study of Gustilo–Anderson grade II and III open fractures, utilising nanocrystalline silver-impregnated dressings as an interface with NPWT reported a favourable deep infection rate of 1 case in 17 (35).

The use of antibiotic-impregnated cement has been proposed as an alternative to intravenous antibiotics for delivery of a high concentration of antibiotics in the vicinity of the injury. Both polymethylmethacrylate (PMMA) and plaster of Paris have been studied as delivery vehicles (36). In a study reporting the outcomes of patients with primary open lower limb fractures randomised to receive either tobramycin-impregnated PMMA beads or intravenous (IV) antibiotics, there were 2 infections in the 24 managed using beads and 2 infections in the 38 managed by IV antibiotics, with no significant difference between the two groups (37). By contrast, a retrospective, non-randomised study of 704 open fractures (35% of which were Grade III) managed with systemic antibiotics with (547) or without (157) tobramycin-impregnated PMMA beads reported infection rates of 17% (26/157) and 4.2% (23/547), respectively. Subanalysis revealed a significant reduction in osteomyelitis in Gustilo–Anderson IIIB fractures (26% to 6.3%) when beads were used in addition to systemic antibiotics (38). Another non-randomised retrospective study reported a significant reduction in deep infection rate (16% (4 in 25) to 4% (2 in 53)) when an antibiotic bead pouch was used in addition to systemic antibiotics (39).

Large animal models have been used to investigate the influence of NPWT on the elution of antibiotics from spacer beads. The use of NPWT concurrently with antibiotic beads may enhance elution of antibiotic from the beads leading to lower locally available concentrations (40, 41). Thus, antibiotic beads should not be used in combination with NPWT.

Conclusion

Whilst NICE previously recommended that NPWT be considered as a temporary dressing for managing open fractures following wound excision, a more recent large randomised clinical trial has shown that the NPWT provides no benefit over standard dressings provided. This finding was supported by the latest Cochrane review of negative pressure wound therapy for open traumatic wounds (42). These data would suggest that provided the other principal recommendations in these Standards are followed, including timely wound excision performed jointly by consultant plastic and orthopaedic surgeons and prompt definitive wound coverage within 72 hours of the injury, the precise dressing used in the intervening period is relatively unimportant. Current evidence suggests that if definitive soft tissue closure of the wound is delayed beyond 3 days the deep infection rate rises steeply and NPWT should not be used to delay definitive closure. This calls into question the strategy of using NPWT for prolonged periods to reduce the reconstructive requirements of the wound. There is low-level evidence to suggest that silver-impregnated dressings or antibiotic-impregnated beads may reduce deep soft tissue and bone infections, respectively, following high-energy open fractures. There is a need for further randomised trials of alternative types of wound dressings and wound management strategies in open fractures. The role of NPWT in managing closed incisions at high risk of wound complications, such as those associated with open fractures, has recently been assessed in a large randomised clinical trial that had shown that the NPWT provides no benefit over standard dressings (42).

References

1. **Glass GE, Barrett SP, Sanderson F, Pearse MF, Nanchahal J.** The microbiological basis for a revised antibiotic regimen in high-energy tibial fractures: preventing deep infections by nosocomial organisms. J Plast Reconstr Aesthet Surg. 2011;64(3):375–80.
2. **National Clinical Guideline Centre (UK).** Fractures (Complex): Assessment and Management. London: National Institute for Health and Care Excellence (UK); 2016 Feb. NG37. https://www.nice.org.uk/guidance/ng37/chapter/Recommendations#hospital-settings
3. **Chariker ME, Jeter KF, Tintle TE, Bottsford JE.** Effective management of incisional and cutaneous fistulae with closed suction wound drainage. Contemp Surg. 1989;34:59–63.

4. **Argenta LC, Morykwas MJ.** Vacuum-assisted closure: a new method for wound control and treatment: clinical experience. Ann Plast Surg. 1997;**38**:563–77.

5. **Morykwas MJ, Argenta LC, Shelton-Brown EI, McGuirt W.** Vacuum-assisted closure: a new method for wound control and treatment: animal studies and basic foundation. Ann Plast Surg. 1997;**38**:553–62.

6. **Saxena V, Hwang C-W, Huang S, Eichbaum Q, Ingber D, Orgill DP.** Vacuum-assisted closure: microdeformations of wounds and cell proliferation. Plast Reconstr Surg. 2004;**114**(5):1086–96.

7. **Kairinos N, Solomons M, Hudson DA.** Negative-pressure wound therapy i: the paradox of negative-pressure wound therapy. Plast Reconstr Surg. 2009;**123**(2):589–98.

8. **Orgill DP, Bayer LR.** Update on negative-pressure wound therapy. Plast Reconstr Surg. 2011;**127**(Suppl.):105S–115S.

9. **Glass GE, Murphy GF, Esmaeili A, Lai L-M, Nanchahal J.** Systematic review of molecular mechanism of action of negative-pressure wound therapy. Br J Surg. 2014;**101**(13):1627–36.

10. **Jones SM, Banwell PE, Shakespeare PG.** interface dressings influence the delivery of topical negative-pressure therapy. Plast Reconstr Surg. 2005;**116**(4):1023–8.

11. **Scherer SS, Pietramaggiori G, Mathews JC, Orgill DP.** Short periodic applications of the vacuum-assisted closure device cause an extended tissue response in the diabetic mouse model. Plast Reconstr Surg. 2009;**124**(5):1458–65.

12. **Dastouri P, Helm DL, Scherer SS, Pietramaggiori G, Younan G, Orgill DP.** Waveform modulation of negative-pressure wound therapy in the murine model. Plast Reconstr Surg. 2011;**127**(4):1460–6.

13. **Glass GE, Nanchahal J.** The methodology of negative pressure wound therapy: separating fact from fiction. J Plast Reconstr Aesthetic Surg. 2012;**65**(8):989–1001.

14. **Kairinos N, Voogd AM, Botha PH, Kotze T, Kahn D, Hudson D,** et al. Negative-pressure wound therapy II: negative-pressure wound therapy and increased perfusion. Just an illusion? Plast Reconstr Surg. 2009;**123**(2):601–12.

15. **Jeffery SL.** Advanced wound therapies in the management of severe military lower limb trauma: a new perspective. Eplasty. 2009 Jan;**9**:e28.

16. **Malmsjö M, Lindstedt S, Ingemansson R.** Influence on pressure transduction when using different drainage techniques and wound fillers (foam and gauze) for negative pressure wound therapy. Int Wound J. 2010;**7**(5):406–12.

17. **Borgquist O, Gustafsson L, Ingemansson R, Malmsjö M.** Micro- and macromechanical effects on the wound bed of negative pressure wound therapy using gauze and foam. Ann Plast Surg. 2010;**64**(6):789–93.

18. **Glass GE, Murphy GRF, Nanchahal J.** Does negative-pressure wound therapy influence subjacent bacterial growth? A systematic review. J Plast Reconstr Aesthetic Surg. 2017;**70**(8):1028–37.

19. **Stinner DJ, Waterman SM, Masini BD, Wenke JC.** Silver dressings augment the ability of negative pressure wound therapy to reduce bacteria in a contaminated open fracture model. J Trauma. 2011;**71**(1 Suppl):S147–50.

20. **Stannard JP, Volgas DA, Stewart R, McGwin G, Alonso JE.** Negative pressure wound therapy after severe open fractures: a prospective randomized study. J Orthop Trauma. 2009;**23**(8):552–7.

21. **Blum ML, Esser M, Richardson M, Eldho P, Rosenfeldt FL.** Negative pressure wound therapy reduces deep infection rate in open tibial fractures. J Orthop Trauma. 2012;**26**(9):499–505.

22. **Costa ML, Achten J, Bruce J, Tutton E, Petrou S, Lamb SE.** Effect of negative pressure wound therapy vs standard wound management on 12-month disability among adults with severe open fracture of the lower limb. The WOLLF Randomized Clinical Trial. JAMA. 2018;**319**(22):2280–8.

23. **Herscovici D, Sanders RW, Scaduto JM, Infante A.** Vacuum-assisted wound closure (VAC therapy) for the management of patients with high energy soft tissue injuries. J Orthop Trauma. 2003;**17**:683–8.

24. **DeFranzo AJ, Argenta LC, Marks MW, Molnar JA, David LR, Webb LX,** et al. The use of vacuum-assisted closure therapy for the treatment of lower-extremity wounds with exposed bone. Plast Reconstr Surg. 2001;**108**(5):1184–91.

25. **Parrett BM, Matros E, Pribaz JJ, Orgill DP.** Lower extremity trauma: trends in the management of soft-tissue reconstruction of open tibia-fibula fractures. Plast Reconstr Surg. 2006;**117**(4):1315–22.

26. **Dedmond BT, Kortesis B, Punger K, Simpson J, Argenta J, Kulp B,** et al. Subatmospheric pressure dressings in the temporary treatment of soft tissue injuries associated with type III open tibial shaft fractures in children. J Pediatr Orthop. 2006;**26**(6):728–32.

27. **Dedmond BT, Kortesis B, Punger K, Simpson J, Argenta J, Kulp B,** et al. The use of negative-pressure wound therapy (NPWT) in the temporary treatment of soft-tissue injuries associated with high-energy open tibial shaft fractures. J Orthop Trauma. 2007;**21**(1):11–7.

28. **Liu DSH, Sofiadellis F, Ashton M, MacGill K, Webb A.** Early soft tissue coverage and negative pressure wound therapy optimises patient outcomes in lower limb trauma. Injury. 2012;**43**(6):772–8.

29. **Bhattacharyya T, Mehta P, Smith M, Pomahac B.** Routine use of wound vacuum-assisted closure does not allow coverage delay for open tibia fractures. Plast Reconstr Surg. 2008;**121**(4):1263–6.

30. **Ashvin R, Ooi A, Ong Y-S, Tan B-K.** Traumatic lower limb injury and microsurgical free flap reconstruction with the use of negative pressure wound therapy: is timing crucial? J Reconstr Microsurg. 2014;**30**(6):427–30.

31. **Kim YH, Hwang KT, Kim JT, Kim SW.** What is the ideal interval between dressing changes during negative pressure wound therapy for open traumatic fractures? J Wound Care. 2015;**24**(11):536–42.

32. **Stannard JP, Volgas DA, McGwin G, Stewart R, Obremsky W, Moore T,** et al. Incisional negative pressure wound therapy after high-risk lower extremity fractures. J Orthop Trauma. 2012;**26**(1):37–42.

33. **Masters JPM, Nanchahal J, Costa ML.** Negative pressure wound therapy and orthopaedic trauma: where are we now? Bone Joint J. 2016;**98**-B(8):1011–13.

34. **Costa ML, Achten J, Knight R, Bruce J, Dutton SJ, Madan J, Dritsaki M, Parsons N, Fernandes M, Jones S, Grant R, Nanchahal J.** Standard wound management versus negative-pressure wound therapy following surgical treatment of major trauma to the lower limb: the WHiST randomized trial. JAMA. 2020;**323**(6):519–26.

35. **Keen JS, Desai PP, Smith CS, Suk M.** Efficacy of hydrosurgical debridement and nanocrystalline silver dressings for infection prevention in type II and III open injuries. Int Wound J. 2012;**9**(1):7–13.

36. **Bowyer GW, Cumberland N.** Antibiotic release from impregnated pellets and beads. J Trauma. 1994;**36**(3):331–5.

37. **Moehring HD, Gravel C, Chapman MW, Olson SA.** Comparison of antibiotic beads and intravenous antibiotics in open fractures. Clin Orthop Relat Res. 2000;**372**:254–61.

38. **Ostermann PA, Henry S., Seligson D.** The role of local antibiotic therapy in the management of compound fractures. Clin Orthop Relat Res. 1993;**29**(5):102–11.

39. **Keating JF, Blachut PA, O'Brien PJ, Meek RN, Broekhuyse H.** Reamed nailing of open tibial fractures: does the antibiotic bead pouch reduce the deep infection rate? J Orthop Trauma. 1996;**10**(5):298–303.

40. **Large TM, Douglas G, Erickson G, Grayson JK.** Effect of negative pressure wound therapy on the elution of antibiotics from polymethylmethacrylate beads in a porcine simulated open femur fracture model. J Orthop Trauma. 2012;**26**(9):506–11.

41. **Stinner DJ, Hsu JR, Wenke JC.** Negative pressure wound therapy reduces the effectiveness of traditional local antibiotic depot in a large complex musculoskeletal wound animal model. J Orthop Trauma. 2012;**26**(9):512–18.

42. **Iheozor-Ejiofor Z, Newton K, Dumville JC, Costa ML, Norman G, Bruce J.** Negative pressure wound therapy for open traumatic wounds. Cochrane Database of Systematic Reviews. 2018;7:CD012522.

Chapter 6

Skeletal Stabilisation

Summary

1. Spanning external fixation is recommended when definitive stabilisation and immediate wound cover are not carried out at the time of primary wound excision (debridement).

2. Spanning external fixation must be stable to prevent fracture site displacement and pain during patient transfer or movement.

3. Fracture patterns, the quantity of bone loss and degree of contamination at injury will determine the most appropriate form of definitive skeletal stabilisation.

4. Internal fixation is safe if there is minimal contamination at the time of injury.

5. If internal fixation is used at any time for stabilisation, it is mandatory for definitive soft tissue cover to be achieved simultaneously.

6. If exchange from spanning external fixation to internal fixation is planned, it is to be done as early as possible (within 3 days).

7. Modern multiplanar and circular fixators are used if there is significant contamination, bone loss, or multilevel fractures of the tibia.

In this chapter we draw upon published evidence and the experience of the authors to provide guidance in stabilisation for open tibial fractures. Most orthopaedic surgeons have, through their training, reached higher levels of proficiency and expertise in methods of internal fixation than with external fixation. The difference reflects the greater number of fractures treated with internal fixation methods. Consequently, we provide a clear rationale for the recommendations made and encourage adoption of the principles described.

Objectives in provisional stabilisation

Provisional stabilisation must control movement between fracture segments and reduce bleeding and pain. Recovery of soft tissues is facilitated by stable fixation, even if provisional (1). Spanning external fixators achieve this objective but the application should factor in the need for additional surgery; in particular, soft tissue reconstruction. Thus, plastic surgeons need to be involved with their orthopaedic colleagues over configurations of external fixators such that the proposed reconstruction of soft tissue defects is unimpeded by the device. Traction or long leg plaster slabs are not recommended after primary debridement.

Various external fixator systems are available for this purpose and are capable of being applied rapidly and easily. There are several fundamental properties that contribute to stable provisional external fixation including component choice, location of pins and overall fixator assembly.

Choosing appropriate fixator components

The generic components are the half-pin (or screw), clamp and rod. Half-pins and rods should be of a large diameter (2). In adults, 5 or 6 mm half-pins should be selected over the smaller 4 mm, whereas in children 4 mm pins are sufficient. Rods should be greater than 10 mm in diameter for adults and rods less than 10 mm, typically 8–9 mm, can be used in children. The bending stiffness of each of these cylindrical components increases exponentially with the fourth power of the radius; by selecting a large diameter half-pin and rod the surgeon can increase the stiffness of the assembled external fixator without need for duplication of components. This simplifies the configuration and facilitates soft tissue reconstruction by leaving a greater space free for unhindered access.

Safe corridors

It was taught previously that the anteromedial surface of the tibia is the safest area to insert a half-pin. Unfortunately, whilst access to drill and insert a pin perpendicular to the subcutaneous surface of the tibia is uncomplicated, the exit point of the drill or half-pin can impinge on either the deep peroneal nerve or anterior tibial artery as both these important structures are situated on the interosseous membrane adjacent to the lateral wall in the proximal three-quarters of the tibia (Figure 6.1). Consequently, we recommend that the pins are inserted 1 cm medial to the crest of the tibia in the sagittal plane (3). Drilling can start perpendicular to the surface of the bone to prevent drill slip but, once the bone surface is entered, the drill should then be brought to a vertical alignment to penetrate the tibia in the sagittal plane. A half-pin inserted in the sagittal plane has the following advantages:

1. It controls displacing forces in the sagittal plane better. For the supine patient, lifting the leg or moving the patient will create displacing forces in this plane from the action of gravity (4).

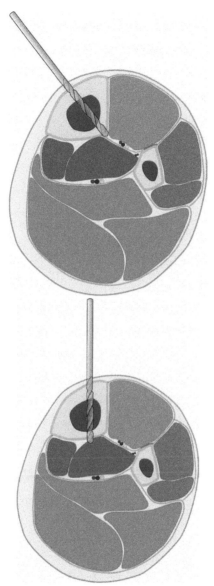

Figure 6.1 (A) The exit point of a drill or half-pin can impinge on either the deep peroneal nerve or anterior tibial artery when inserted perpendicular to the medial subcutaneous surface. (B) A sagittal half-pin has a buffer of the deep posterior muscles in most of the length of the tibia before the posterior tibial neurovascular bundle is placed at risk.

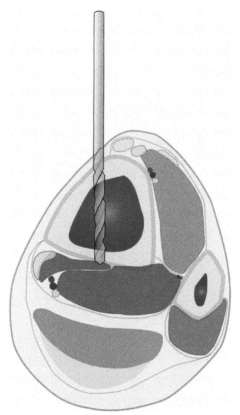

Figure 6.2 In the distal third of the tibia, the deep posterior muscles become tendons but continue to shield the neurovascular bundle as this shifts towards the medial side.

2. It allows for connecting an anterior bar across the pins, thereby leaving both medial and lateral sides of the leg free for soft tissue reconstructive procedures.

3. The exit point of the drill or half-pin is buffered by the deep posterior muscles of the leg in the proximal three-quarters of the leg before the posterior tibial neurovascular bundle is at risk. In the distal quarter, these muscles transition to tendons but continue to shield the neurovascular bundle as it locates towards the medial side (Figure 6.2).

Pin placement in the foot has to factor in the local anatomy. Pins from the medial or lateral side into the calcaneum (or transcalcaneal pins in this area) can be inserted safely if sited at the junction of the posterior quarter and anterior three-quarters of a line subtended between the tip of the malleolus and postero-inferior point of the calcaneal tuberosity (Figure 6.3). Blunt dissection down to

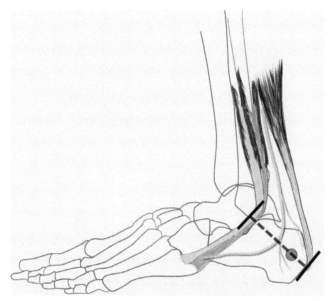

Figure 6.3 The junction of the posterior quarter and anterior three-quarters of a line subtended between the tip of the malleolus and postero-inferior point of the calcaneal tuberosity is a safe entry point for a half-pin.

bone is essential after incision in order to avoid injury to either the medial or lateral calcaneal branches of the posterior tibial nerve. Using a drill sleeve also protects against iatrogenic injury to important neurovascular structures (5–7).

In addition to a pin in the calcaneum, a second level of fixation is needed if the configuration of the external fixator is to span the ankle. A single transcalcaneal pin is insufficient on its own to provide optimum stability across the ankle joint. The locus for the second pin includes the talar neck, base of first metatarsal, or cuboid.

The half-pin placed into the neck of the talus is inserted halfway between the tip of the medial malleolus and tuberosity of the navicular. Centring the drill is facilitated by 'walking' the drill tip anteriorly and posteriorly on the medial surface of the neck until a central position is identified. If this pin is inserted from the lateral side, the contours of the neck of the talus are palpated easily if the entire forefoot is adducted (7). The advantages of using the talar neck as a site for pin insertion are that it allows a pin diameter as large as that used in the tibia (5–6 mm) and the density of bone in this area provides excellent grip—both contribute to the stability of the external fixator.

Half-pins into the base of the first metatarsal should be smaller in diameter (3.5–4.5 mm) in order to avoid iatrogenic fracture after removal and need to be inserted obliquely and not transversely to avoid injury to the dorsalis pedis continuation of the anterior tibial artery (8). The cuboid on the lateral side of the foot accepts 5–6 mm pins but the density of cancellous bone here does not cater for as secure a grip as that of the neck of the talus.

If a knee-spanning configuration is required for open fractures of the proximal third of the tibia, pins placed in an anterolateral direction in the middle-third of the femur have a biomechanical advantage and are safe to insert (9).

Assembling the fixator for stability and facility for soft tissue reconstruction

The simplest **stable** configuration is assembled.

For middle third fractures, where knee or ankle-spanning fixators are not needed (unless an injury exists in the femur or foot, respectively), a single anterior bar is all that is required. Four pins with two in each segment will suffice provided the pins are placed near to and far from the fracture within each segment (the near–far principle). This spread of pins in each segment exerts an advantageous grip but the caveat is to avoid placing pins within exposed tibia or within the zone of injury.

A simple way to achieve this four pin-single bar assembly is to insert the most proximal and most distal pins first and connect the single bar between them. Traction is applied across the fracture to achieve approximate alignment and the clamps then tightened. The additional two pins closer to the fracture are then inserted through additional clamps attached to the same rod; some improvement to the quality of reduction is possible when these pins are introduced. Such a construct achieves the 'near–far' half-pin placement with regard to the fracture site and produces good control of proximal and distal segments of the fracture (Figure 6.4A–D).

When the fracture is situated in the distal third of the tibia, there may be room for a single pin in the distal segment or none at all, e.g. in open fractures of the tibial plafond. In these circumstances, crossing the ankle joint provides additional stability as the short distal tibial portion together with the foot constitute the 'distal segment'. Pin placement in the foot and ankle requires some thought; the calcaneum, first metatarsal, neck of talus, and cuboid can be used. Two separate pins in the foot provide far better control than a single transcalcaneal pin. Again, control of sagittal plane forces is more important as ankle movement occurs in this plane, as does the displacing effect of gravity during patient movement or transfer. A single half-pin in the calcaneum used with a talar neck or base of metatarsal pin is a good combination. The delta configuration assembled with a transcalcaneal pin and metatarsal pin is a simple stable construct as is the delta

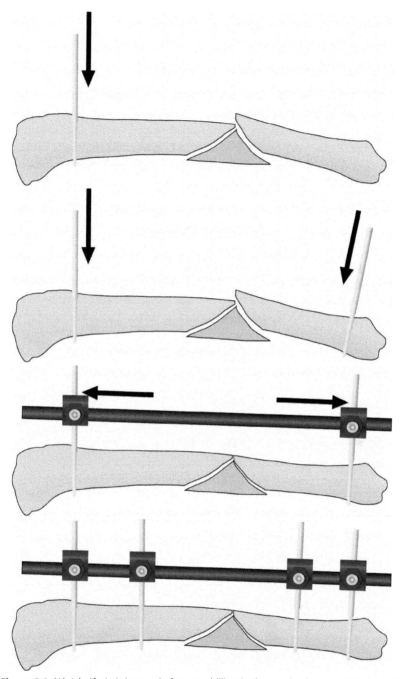

Figure 6.4 (A) A half-pin is inserted after pre-drilling in the proximal segment. This pin is placed 1 cm medial to the crest of the tibia and in the sagittal plane. It helps if this is also perpendicular to the axis of the tibia in the lateral view. (B) A second half-pin is inserted in a similar position but in the distal segment. (C) Traction is applied to provisionally reduce the fracture between the two pins above and the clamps tightened. (D) Because these two pins are in the 'far–far' positions with respect to the fracture, some direct manipulation of the fracture for improved alignment is possible (as it is an open fracture) before the 'near–near' pins are inserted off clamps attached to the same rod.

frame from the single calcaneal half-pin and talar neck pin. The first assembly involves oblique bars across both sides of the distal tibia which may impede soft tissue reconstruction from both sides (Figure 6.5), whereas the second assembly can be constructed on either the medial or lateral side of the leg in anticipation of soft tissue surgery from the opposite side (Figure 6.6A–F). A 'kickstand' bar attached posteriorly elevates the limb and the heel from the bed and is helpful in protection against decubitus ulcers and limb swelling (Figure 6.7) (10, 11).

Definitive stabilisation

The primary objectives in treatment are to achieve union without infection and through as few additional operative procedures as possible. Both internal and external fixation techniques have their place. Variables that are considered when deciding on the type of definitive fixation include the fracture pattern, degree and type of initial contamination, timing of definitive soft tissue cover, and the presence of dead space after wound excision. Systematic reviews that

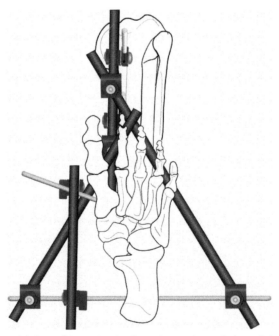

Figure 6.5 An axial view of a construct using a transcalcaneal pin and single first metatarsal pin. This is a stable construct but has the disadvantage—in the context of open fractures of the tibia—in that one oblique rod between tibia and calcaneal pin has to be disassembled to allow access for any plastic surgical intervention on that side.

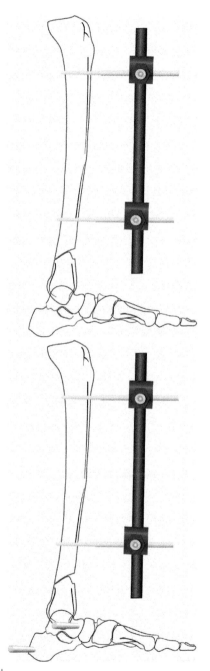

Figure 6.6 Continued

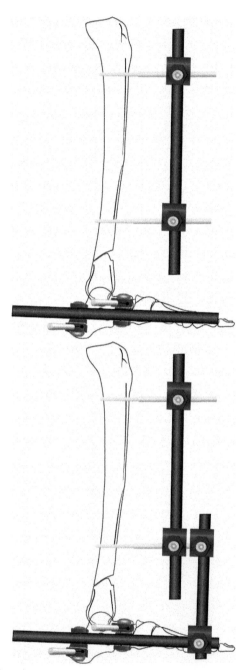

Figure 6.6 Continued

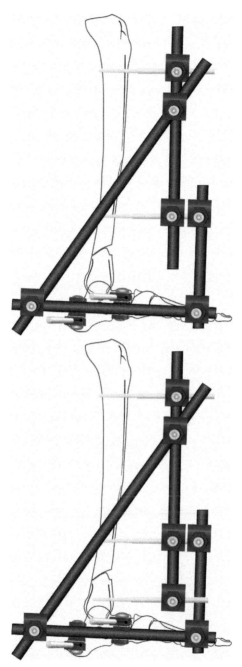

Figure 6.6 (A–6F) The following sequence (6A–6F) shows a construct that is based on a single calcaneal half-pin and talar neck pin for the distal segment. Both calcaneal and talar neck pin can be inserted from the medial or lateral side thereby allowing access for plastic surgery from the contralateral position. When done after collaborative planning with the plastic surgeon, this provides a stable construct that requires no disassembly for subsequent soft tissue reconstruction. Sometimes the distal segment of the tibia is sufficiently large to allow addition of a half-pin into it without jeopardising the nearby soft tissues (6F).

have attempted guidance in this area have been hampered by the randomised trials using treatment devices that are now outdated or have included studies with poor precision (12, 13). Future studies may provide clearer advice (14).

Anatomy of the fracture

Fracture patterns are strong determinants of the definitive method of stabilisation: diaphyseal injuries with minimal bone loss are suited to locked intramedullary nails, whereas articular fractures are held well by plates and screws. Injuries with significant bone loss, articular fractures with comminution especially at the metaphyseal level, complex multilevel fractures, and those with associated ankle or knee joint instability are suitable for circular external fixation.

Degree of contamination

Internal fixation should not be used in injuries highly contaminated with road grit, soil, or sewage.

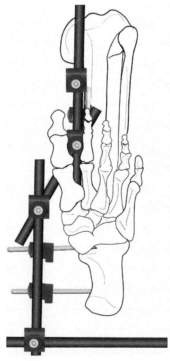

Figure 6.7 An axial view showing how a 'kickstand' can be constructed simply by adding an additional bar across from the posterior aspect of the bar connecting the calcaneal and talar neck pins. This has the advantages of elevation and prevention of decubitus ulcers on the heel as well as protection of any local tissue or free tissue transfers performed by plastic surgeons.

Timing of definitive cover

The National Institute for Health and Care Excellence (NICE) recommends that if internal fixation is used, it is essential that definitive soft tissue cover is achieved at the same time. Delayed cover over internal fixation leads to increased and unacceptable infection rates (15–18).

Internal fixation can be used safely in open injuries which, after wound excision (debridement), can be closed by simple suture of the wound (typically Gustilo–Anderson grades I and II) (19). If wound closure requires a local or free flap and the fracture has little bone loss or contamination, internal fixation carries low rates of infection as long as definitive soft tissue closure using well-vascularised tissue is achieved at the same time. Such situations occur when both orthopaedic and plastic surgeons decide that definitive skeletal stabilisation and cover can be accomplished then and there and safely. In that scenario, the entire operative procedure is carried out as a formal second intervention; this would involve new instruments, a re-prep and re-drape of the limb, and the surgical team changing into fresh attire. Whilst direct evidence to support this two-procedure single-stage event is absent, open injuries that are excised (debrided) and lavaged of gross or even microscopic contaminants will render all instruments and drapes used unsterile without exception.

In contrast, if provisional external fixation is used and wound closure delayed, conversion to internal fixation should proceed cautiously. The risks associated with conversion from provisional spanning external fixation to internal fixation have not been quantified. Recommendations that intervals of 4–28 days are 'safe' are quoted but intramedullary canal contamination from pin sites is an early phenomenon and infection from one pin site tracking along the canal to reach the remainder of the cavity does occur (20–23). If conversion from external to internal fixation is planned, we recommended that this be achieved within 72 hours of the primary wound excision (debridement) (this implies that it is performed usually at the second-look procedure) and that definitive soft tissue cover is achieved at the same time. If this window of opportunity for conversion is missed, consideration should be given to definitive management with modern multiplanar or circular external fixators.

Degree and location of soft tissue and bone loss

Current techniques for dealing with bone loss include the creation of new bone by distraction osteogenesis (the Ilizarov method) or autogenous bone grafting following use of a cement spacer in the defect (the Masquelet method) (24–26). The former technique is well established and reliable; if the fracture characteristics are such that this method is to be employed in reconstruction of the limb, circular external fixation or a rail-type external fixator will be a better choice for definitive stabilisation. Smaller losses of bone—usually cuneiform in shape rather than segmental defects—can be treated by a planned autogenous bone grafting later; here internal or external fixation can be the definitive stabilisation depending on the level of the fracture and contamination at injury.

Dead space and management

In severe open injuries, tissue loss occurs either primarily (direct consequence of the injury where fragments or segments of bone are extruded and left at the scene of trauma) or secondarily after wound excision (debridement). In both, there is a resulting defect that becomes filled with haematoma. This haematoma-filled space can be prevented through the use of negative pressure wound dressings, antibiotic-impregnated cement spacers and, in some instances, performing an acute shortening of the limb with the intention of restoring length at a later stage. Acute shortening, if used for dead space management, may influence the choice of stabilisation device as it is more common for a circular or rail-type fixator to be used in this scenario as it then can be utilised for the subsequent limb lengthening (27).

Dead space is often thought of as a cavity but any structure unable to provide some resistance to bacterial proliferation within or on itself—non-viable tissue, haematoma, internal fixation devices—behaves as dead space. For these reasons, meticulous wound excision (debridement), pervention of cavities, avoidance of internal fixation in highly contaminated injuries, and early definitive soft tissue cover remain guiding principles for treating open fractures of the tibia.

Conclusion

Stable spanning external fixation is applied at the time of primary wound excision (debridement) if definitive fracture fixation is not performed. The choice of components and the fixator configuration should resist displacing forces at the fracture site during patient transfer or with patient movement. The applied fixator should enable the proposed soft tissue reconstruction to be carried out without impediment.

If definitive soft tissue cover can be provided at primary wound excision (debridement) and wound contamination is minimal, internal fixation is a suitable choice for definitive stabilisation. If soft tissue cover is delayed, there is significant contamination, or for complex fracture patterns with bone loss, modern multiplanar or circular fixators are more appropriate. In a combined orthoplastic approach, bone and soft tissue reconstruction strategies are planned together; decisions are made that enable both to be carried out with each facilitating the other.

References

1. **Camuso MR.** Far-forward fracture stabilization: external fixation versus splinting. J Am Acad Orthop Surg. 2006;**14**(10):S118–23.

2. **Giotakis N, Narayan B.** Stability with unilateral external fixation in the tibia. Strategies Trauma Limb Reconstr. 2007;**2**(1):13–20.

3. **Nayagam S.** Safe corridors in external fixation: the lower leg (tibia, fibula, hindfoot and forefoot). Strategies Trauma Limb Reconstr. 2007;**2**(2-3):105–10.

4. **Behrens F, Johnson W.** Unilateral external fixation methods to increase and reduce frame stiffness. Clin Orthop Relat Res. 1989;**241**:48–56.

5. **Thomson CM, Esparon T, Rea PM, Jamal B.** Monoaxial external fixation of the calcaneus: an anatomical study assessing the safety of monoaxial pin insertion. Injury. 2016;**47**(10):2091–6.

6. **Casey D, McConnell T, Parekh S, Tornetta PI.** Percutaneous pin placement in the medial calcaneus: is anywhere safe? J Orthop Trauma. 2002;**16**(1):26–9.

7. **Santi MD, Botte MJ.** External fixation of the calcaneus and talus: an anatomical study for safe pin insertion. J Orthop Trauma. 1996;**10**(7):487–91.

8. **Barrett MO, Wade AM, Della Rocca GJ, Crist BD, Anglen JO.** The safety of forefoot metatarsal pins in external fixation of the lower extremity. JBone Joint Surg. 2008;**90**(3):560–4.

9. **Mercer D, Firoozbakhsh K, Prevost M, Mulkey P, DeCoster TA, Schenck R.** Stiffness of knee-spanning external fixation systems for traumatic knee dislocations: a biomechanical study. J Orthop Trauma. 2010;**24**(11):693–6.

10. **Roukis TS, Landsman AS, Weinberg SA, Leone E.** Use of a hybrid 'kickstand' external fixator for pressure relief after soft-tissue reconstruction of heel defects. J Foot Ankle Surg. 2003;**42**(4):240–3.

11. **Castro-Aragon OE, Rapley JH, Trevino SG.** The use of a kickstand modification for the prevention of heel decubitus ulcers in trauma patients with lower extremity external fixation. J Orthop Trauma. 2009;**23**(2):145–7.

12. **Bhandari MGGH, Swiontkowski MF, Schemitsch EH.** Treatment of open fractures of the shaft of the tibia: a systematic overview and meta-analysis. J Bone Joint Surg. 2001;**83B**(1):62–8.

13. **Foote CJ, Guyatt GH, Vignesh KN, Mundi R, Chaudhry H, Heels-Ansdell D,** et al. Which surgical treatment for open tibial shaft fractures results in the fewest reoperations? A network meta-analysis. Clin Orthop Relat Res. 2015;**473**(7):2179–92.

14. **O'Toole R, Gary J, Reider L, Bosse M, Gordon W, Hutson J,** et al. A prospective randomized trial to assess fixation strategies for severe open tibia fractures: modern ring external fixators versus internal fixation (FIXIT Study). J Orthop Trauma. 2017;**31**:S10–17.

15. **Naique SB, Pearse M, Nanchahal J.** Management of severe open tibial fractures: the need for combined orthopaedic and plastic surgical treatment in specialist centres. J Bone Joint Surg Br. 2006;**88-B**(3):351–7.

16. **Gopal S, Majumder S, Batchelor A, Knight S, Boer PD, Smith R.** Fix and flap: the radical orthopaedic and plastic treatment of severe open fractures of the tibia. J Bone Joint Surg Br 2000;**82-B**:959–66.

17. **Yokoyama K, Uchino M, Nakamura K, Ohtsuka H, Suzuki T, Boku T**, et al. Risk factors for deep infection in secondary intramedullary nailing after external fixation for open tibial fractures. Injury. 2006;**37**(6):554–60.

18. **National Institute for Health and Care Excellence (NICE) GDG.** Open fractures: National Institute for Health and Care Excellence; February 2016. https://www.nice.org.uk/guidance/ng37/chapter/Recommendations#hospital-settings

19. **Jenkinson RJ, Kiss A, Johnson S, Stephen DJ, Kreder HJ.** Delayed wound closure increases deep-infection rate associated with lower-grade open fractures: a propensity-matched cohort study. J Bone Joint Surg Am. 2014;**96**(5):380–6.

20. **Clasper JC, Cannon LB, Stapley SA, Taylor VM, Watkins PE.** Fluid accumulation and the rapid spread of bacteria in the pathogenesis of external fixator pin track infection. Injury. 2001;**32**(5):377–81.

21. **Clasper JC, Parker SJ, Simpson AH, Watkins PE.** Contamination of the medullary canal following pin-tract infection. J Orthop Res. 1999;**17**(6):947–52.

22. **Bhandari M, Zlowodzki M, Tornetta PI, Schmidt A, Templeman DC.** Intramedullary nailing following external fixation in femoral and tibial shaft fractures. J Orthop Trauma. 2005;**19**(2):140–4.

23. **Metsemakers WJ, Handojo K, Reynders P, Sermon A, Vanderschot P, Nijs S.** Individual risk factors for deep infection and compromised fracture healing after intramedullary nailing of tibial shaft fractures: a single centre experience of 480 patients. Injury. 2015;**46**(4):740–5.

24. **Giannoudis PV, Faour O, Goff T, Kanakaris N, Dimitriou R.** Masquelet technique for the treatment of bone defects: tips-tricks and future directions. Injury. 2011;**42**(6):591–8.

25. **Lowenberg DW, Buntic RF, Buncke GM, Parrett BM.** Long-term results and costs of muscle flap coverage with Ilizarov bone transport in lower limb salvage. J Orthop Trauma. 2013;**27**(10):576–81.

26. **Rozbruch SR, Weitzman A, Watson JT, Freudigman P, Katz H, Ilizarov S.** Simultaneous treatment of tibial bone and soft-tissue defects with the Ilizarov method. J Orthop Trauma. 2006;**20**(3):194–202.

27. **Lavini F, Dall'Oca C, Bartolozzi P.** Bone transport and compression-distraction in the treatment of bone loss of the lower limbs. Injury. 2010;**41**(11):1191–5.

Chapter 7

Timing of Soft Tissue Reconstruction

Summary

1. Early definitive soft tissue cover is associated with better outcomes, including reduced deep infection rates.

2. Definitive soft tissue cover should be performed either at the same time as wound excision or within 72 hours of injury.

3. Free flap reconstruction is best performed on scheduled lists by experienced, dedicated senior surgical teams following adequate preparation of the patient. This must include optimum physiology and planning. CT scanning with an angiogram may help with planning of osteo-synthese as well as the free flap. This should be undertaken in a specialist centre offering the full spectrum of orthoplastic services.

4. If internal fixation is used, definitive soft tissue cover should be performed at the same time.

Introduction

Soft tissue cover of a meticulously and comprehensively excised (debrided) wound is the cornerstone of achieving infection-free fracture union (1–3). Before the significance of the soft tissue structures surrounding the fractured bone was recognised, reconstruction of the soft tissue defect was consigned to the 'delayed' phase (4). Early 'open wound' management methods were associated with extremely high rates of complications, for example, 40% develop osteomyelitis and 30% non-union (5). Early soft tissue cover may reduce the risk of bacterial contamination and biofilm development. The role of early coverage of open tibial fractures using muscle flaps to prevent deep infection was recognised as early as 1977 (6) and this paradigm was developed subsequently using free flaps (7).

Current National Institute for Health and Care Excellence (NICE) Guidelines advocate definitive coverage within 72 hours if this cannot be performed at the time of primary wound excision (8). Provided comprehensive wound excision has been achieved, early definitive soft tissue coverage of open fractures is associated with reduced free flap failure and deep infection rates. Moreover, delay leads to tissue oedema, peri-vascular fibrosis, and an increased risk of venous thrombosis, making the surgery more challenging technically.

A number of studies have investigated the effect of timing of soft tissue coverage. Whilst the definition of early and delayed wound closure varied between studies, the literature suggests that the best outcomes are achieved when the wounds are covered at the earliest opportunity.

Various historic studies found that lengthy delays were associated with dramatically poorer outcomes. A retrospective series of over 500 cases demonstrated that free tissue transfer performed within 3 days, rather than 3 days to 3 months of injury, was associated with improved flap survival (0.75 vs 12%) and reduced infection rates (1.5 vs 17.5%) (7). A review of muscle flaps in grade IIIB open tibial fractures found that patients with flap cover within 10 days spent less time in hospital and had a deep infection rate of 18% compared with 69% in the delayed groups combined (9).

A group reviewing their outcome of 83 flap reconstructions in 64 patients found that the rate of deep infection associated with metal implants was significantly lower in the early coverage group (<5 days) compared with the delayed group, as were the rates of free flap failure and local flap partial necrosis (10). Another study of 105 patients who underwent free muscle flap reconstruction for open tibial fractures found that flaps performed between 1 and 7 days post-injury were associated with a lower overall complication rate of 31% compared with 39% in the >42 days group and 47% in the 8–42 days group, whilst the time to fracture union was 2.4 compared with 6.5 versus 6.2 months, respectively (11). Early coverage with fasciocutaneous flaps has also been found to be beneficial. In a study of 38 patients with Gustilo–Anderson IIIB fractures in whom fasciocutaneous flaps was the predominant reconstructive option, the infection rate was found to be significantly lower in patients who had coverage within 7 days of injury (12.5%) compared with coverage at 7 or more days (53%); furthermore, there was no evidence of a relationship between flap type and infection rate (12) Similar improved outcomes for patients undergoing definitive soft tissue reconstruction within 1 week have been reported by other groups (13–17).

Further studies that attempted to assess the risk of delay suggest that wounds should be covered at the earliest opportunity. Using multivariate analysis, a study of 69 tibial fractures found that the odds of flap-related complications and infection increased by 11% and 16%, respectively, for each day after 7 days post-injury (18). A retrospective study of 137 type III fractures also used multivariate analysis and found that a delay of more than 5 days to wound coverage was an independent predictor of infection, with an odds ratio of 7.39 (19).

The effect of even shorter delays was reported in a review of 105 consecutive free flap reconstructions for severe open lower limb trauma in 103 patients (20). The outcomes of patients reconstructed within 3 days of injury were compared with those beyond 7 days. The latter group had significantly increased rates of wound infection prior to free flap reconstruction, flap re-operation, deep metal infection (4.2 vs 28.6%, p < 0.05) and osteomyelitis (4.2 vs 21.4%, p < 0.05). In cases of exposed metalwork, free flap transfer beyond 1 day significantly increased the flap failure rate (0 vs 50%) and was associated with a greater overall number of surgical procedures as well as a longer hospital stay.

Immediate versus staged reconstruction

The concept of the 'fix and flap' approach where skeletal fixation and soft tissue reconstruction are undertaken in a single stage was introduced with the aim of achieving earlier fracture union and minimising flap failure and deep infection rates (21). A retrospective review of patients with grade IIIB or IIIC fractures compared the effect of timing of reconstruction on deep infection rates (22). In the first group, primary closure was achieved in a single 'fix and flap' procedure, comprising wound excision and skeletal stabilisation with a muscle flap. The second and third groups underwent immediate wound excision and internal fixation but soft tissue cover was achieved between 48 and 72 hours, and over 72 hours, respectively. The times to fracture union (28.8, 35.3, and 43.1 weeks, respectively) were shorter in the 'fix and flap' group. Another group reviewed grade III fractures in 73 consecutive patients and compared those who underwent definitive fixation and immediate coverage against patients who had staged operations. The deep infection rate in the immediate group was only 4.2% compared with 34.6% in the staged group (23). Similarly, a retrospective study of 89 Gustilo–Anderson IIIB fractures found that delayed soft tissue reconstruction was associated with osteomyelitis in 60% and flap failure in 23% compared with 4% for both in the immediate group (24). A prospective cohort study of 29 consecutive patients with IIIB or IIIC fractures compared immediate with delayed reconstruction (after a mean delay of 4.4 days) with a mean follow up of 47 months. In the delayed group, time to full unprotected weight bearing (9.6 months vs 5 months), time to definitive union (11.6 months vs 5.6 months), the number of operations (3.9 vs 1.6), and the deep infection rate (4/15 vs 0/14) were all significantly higher (25).

Conclusion

It is not possible to be prescriptive as to the exact number of days post-injury that soft tissue cover should be achieved as it depends on the individual circumstances of the injury and patient. For example, in the polytrauma setting, life must come before limb. Whilst immediate soft tissue reconstruction, as implied by the 'fix and flap' protocol, may seem to be the ideal, complex surgery, especially those requiring microsurgical free tissue transfer, should be undertaken only once the patient has been stabilised, adequately prepared, and investigated, and should be performed under elective conditions by dedicated senior surgeons working within experienced orthoplastic teams in specialist centres. This is balanced by the increasing risk of deep infection and technical difficulties encountered as the perivascular soft tissues become more oedematous, friable, and eventually fibrotic. Therefore, soft tissue reconstruction should be performed at the earliest safe opportunity to maximise the chances of long-term success. The current NICE guidance (8), based on the available evidence, recommends that if definitive reconstruction is not performed at the time of wound excision, it should be achieved within 72 hours of injury unless patient factors dictate otherwise. Internal fixation should only be performed if definitive soft tissue reconstruction is achieved at the same time.

References

1. **Cierny G, 3rd, Byrd HS, Jones RE.** Primary versus delayed soft tissue coverage for severe open tibial fractures. A comparison of results. Clin Orthop Relat Res. 1983(**178**):54–63.

2. **Edwards CC, Simmons SC, Browner BD, Weigel MC.** Severe open tibial fractures. Results treating 202 injuries with external fixation. Clin Orthop Relat Res. 1988(**230**):98–115.

3. **Gustilo RB, Anderson JT.** Prevention of infection in the treatment of one thousand and twenty-five open fractures of long bones: retrospective and prospective analyses. J Bone Joint Surg Am. 1976;**58**(4):453–8.

4. **Chacha PB.** Salvage of severe open fractures of the tibia that might have required amputation. Injury. 1974;**6**(2):154–72.

5. **Byrd HS, Spicer TE, Cierney G,** 3rd. Management of open tibial fractures. Plast Reconstr Surg. 1985;**76**(5):719–30.

6. **Ger R.** Muscle transposition for treatment and prevention of chronic post-traumatic osteomyelitis of the tibia. J Bone Joint Surg Am. 1977;**59**(6):784–91.

7. **Godina M.** Early microsurgical reconstruction of complex trauma of the extremities. Plast Reconstr Surg. 1986;**78**(3):285–92.

8. **National Institute for Health and Care Excellence (NICE).** NICE guidance: fractures (complex). 2016. https://www.nice.org.uk/guidance/ng37/evidence

9. **Fischer MD, Gustilo RB, Varecka TF.** The timing of flap coverage, bone-grafting, and intramedullary nailing in patients who have a fracture of the tibial shaft with extensive soft-tissue injury. J Bone Joint Surg Am. 1991;73(9):1316–22.

10. **Lo CH, Leung M, Baillieu C, Chong EW, Cleland H.** Trauma centre experience: flap reconstruction of traumatic lower limb injuries. ANZ J Surg. 2007;77(8): 690–4.

11. **Rinker B, Amspacher JC, Wilson PC, Vasconez HC.** Subatmospheric pressure dressing as a bridge to free tissue transfer in the treatment of open tibia fractures. Plast Reconstr Surg. 2008;121(5):1664–73.

12. **Bhattacharyya T, Mehta P, Smith M, Pomahac B.** Routine use of wound vacuum-assisted closure does not allow coverage delay for open tibia fractures. Plast Reconstr Surg. 2008;121(4):1263–6.

13. **Caudle RJ, Stern PJ.** Severe open fractures of the tibia. J Bone Joint Surg Am. 1987;69(6):801–7.

14. **Choudry U, Moran S, Karacor Z.** Soft-tissue coverage and outcome of Gustilo grade IIIB midshaft tibia fractures: a 15-year experience. Plast Reconstr Surg. 2008;122(2):479–85.

15. **Olesen UK, Juul R, Bonde CT, Moser C, McNally M, Jensen LT,** et al. A review of forty five open tibial fractures covered with free flaps. Analysis of complications, microbiology and prognostic factors. Int Orthop. 2015;39(6):1159–66.

16. **Rezzadeh KS, Nojan M, Buck A, Li A, Vardanian A, Crisera C,** et al. The use of negative pressure wound therapy in severe open lower extremity fractures: identifying the association between length of therapy and surgical outcomes. J Surg Res. 2015;199(2):726–31.

17. **Hou Z, Irgit K, Strohecker KA, Matzko ME, Wingert NC, DeSantis JG,** et al. Delayed flap reconstruction with vacuum-assisted closure management of the open IIIB tibial fracture. J Trauma. 2011;71(6):1705–8.

18. **D'Alleyrand JC, Manson TT, Dancy L, Castillo RC, Bertumen JB, Meskey T,** et al. Is time to flap coverage of open tibial fractures an independent predictor of flap-related complications? J Orthop Trauma. 2014;28(5):288–93.

19. **Lack WD, Karunakar MA, Angerame MR, Seymour RB, Sims S, Kellam JF,** et al. Type III open tibia fractures: immediate antibiotic prophylaxis minimizes infection. J Orthop Trauma. 2015;29(1):1–6.

20. **Liu DS, Sofiadellis F, Ashton M, MacGill K, Webb A.** Early soft tissue coverage and negative pressure wound therapy optimises patient outcomes in lower limb trauma. Injury. 2012;43(6):772–8.

21. **Gopal S, Majumder S, Batchelor AG, Knight SL, De Boer P, Smith RM.** Fix and flap: the radical orthopaedic and plastic treatment of severe open fractures of the tibia. J Bone Joint Surg Br. 2000;82(7):959–66.

22. **Gopal S, Giannoudis PV, Murray A, Matthews SJ, Smith RM.** The functional outcome of severe, open tibial fractures managed with early fixation and flap coverage. J Bone Joint Surg Br. 2004;86(6):861–7.

23. **Mathews JA, Ward J, Chapman TW, Khan UM, Kelly MB.** Single-stage orthoplastic reconstruction of Gustilo-Anderson grade III open tibial fractures greatly reduces infection rates. Injury. 2015;46(11):2263–6.

24. **Bellidenty L, Chastel R, Pluvy I, Pauchot J, Tropet Y.** [Emergency free flap in reconstruction of the lower limb. Thirty-five years of experience]. Ann Chir Plast Esthet. 2014;**59**(1):35–41.

25. **Hertel R, Lambert SM, Muller S, Ballmer FT, Ganz R.** On the timing of soft-tissue reconstruction for open fractures of the lower leg. Arch Orthop Trauma Surg. 1999;**119**(1–2):7–12.

Chapter 8

Soft Tissue Reconstruction

Summary

1. All open fractures must be covered with well-vascularised soft tissue within 72 hours of the injury to achieve infection-free bony union.

2. If internal fixation is used, definitive soft tissue coverage should be achieved at the same time.

3. Dressings, including negative pressure wound therapy, can temporise for cover following wound excision but should not be used as a substitute for definitive flap coverage.

4. The medial fasciotomy incision is used to raise local fasciocutaneous flaps or to access the posterior tibial vessels for microsurgical anastomosis in free flap reconstruction.

5. Local fasciocutaneous flaps are usually best reserved for patients with relatively low-energy injuries and a limited zone of injury.

6. Experimental data suggest that coverage with muscle leads to improved healing of fractures. However, there is currently little clinical evidence to support the use of one form of soft tissue cover over another for open fractures of the lower limb. When choosing a flap, careful consideration should be given to donor site morbidity.

Types of soft tissue coverage

Soft tissue coverage may be in the form of local or free flaps, and may comprise muscle, fasciocutaneous tissues, or both. Flap selection depends on multiple factors, including the size and location of the defect following wound excision, availability of flaps, and donor site morbidity. Additionally, there is increasing evidence to support the biological contribution of soft tissue flaps in fracture repair by providing the optimal availability of growth factors as well as a source of regenerative stem and progenitor cells (1).

Planning and incisions

We recommend that the incisions used to raise local fasciocutaneous flaps as well as to access vessels for microsurgical anastomosis of free flaps are based on the medial fasciotomy incision (see Figure 3.1, Chapter 3). The same incision will have been used to provide access for wound excision of the open fracture. This minimises the risk of damaging the perforating vessels that supply the overlying skin whilst providing good access to the posterior tibial vessels. The medial incision is placed 1.5 cm posterior to the medial subcutaneous border of the tibia and lies anterior to the posterior tibial artery. Placement of the incision too anteriorly risks exposure of the tibia in the tense, swollen limb. Conversely, if the incision is too posterior, it will lie behind the fasciocutaneous perforators and hence preclude the use of flaps based on them. Therefore, accurate placement is essential and we recommend marking the anatomical landmarks before making the incisions.

Local flaps

In general, local flaps are best suited for defects with a limited zone of injury from low-energy trauma. The flap chosen should lie outside the zone of injury to minimise complications such as partial or complete necrosis. A common cause of failure is raising fasciocutaneous flaps in areas where the skin has been degloved. Care must also be taken to ensure the fracture is covered and the entire flap survives. Partial or tip necrosis is equivalent to complete flap failure as this would mean conversion back to an open fracture with the associated risks of poor outcomes. Therefore, local flaps should be reserved for relatively low-energy injuries where the zone of injury is limited. For higher energy injuries and those with degloving free tissue transfer is necessary.

Local fasciocutaneous flaps

An understanding of the topography of lower limb angiosomes together with accurate mapping of perforating vessels has enabled the reliable use of local fasciocutaneous flaps (2, 3) (Figure 8.1). The most commonly used are based on the septocutaneous perforators that arise reliably from the posterior tibial artery with at least one vena commitans on the medial aspect of the tibia (4–7). Proximally based flaps extending as far distal as the '15 cm perforator' (located about 15 cm proximal to the tip of the medial malleolus) can be raised reliably, especially if incorporating the saphenous vein and the artery that runs with the saphenous nerve about 1 cm behind. The anterior border of the flap lies 1.5 cm posterior and medial to the medial subcutaneous border of the tibia, coinciding with the medial fasciotomy incision. The posterior margin can extend to the

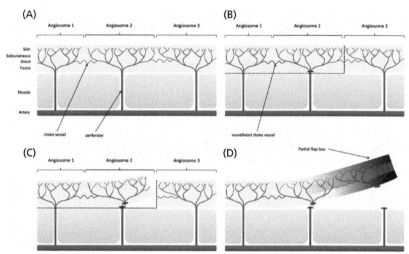

Figure 8.1 The angiosome concept: an angiosome is a block of tissue (skin, muscle, bone, or a combination) supplied by an artery and the accompanying veins. It can survive when isolated on this pedicle. (a) The posterior tibial artery is an example of an axial artery along which a series of perforators arise to supply the overlying fascia and skin. Each perforator supplies an angiosome. (b) When the perforator to an angiosome is occluded, 'choke' or 'variable resistance' vessels, which connect to the adjacent angiosome, dilate to maintain the blood supply of the affected angiosome. (c) Usually, a perforator will only reliably perfuse one adjacent angiosome through opening of the intervening choke vessel. Therefore, it is possible to raise a fasciocutaneous flap comprising two angiosomes based on a single perforator to cover local defects. (d) However, attempts to capture more than a single adjacent angiosome risk necrosis of the distal part of the flap.

posterior midline, taking care to avoid injuring the sural nerve. The deep fascia is included within the flap to protect the delicate vascular plexus that lies just superficial to the fascia. It is important to preserve the filmy vascularised tissue overlying the proximal part of the Achilles tendon so as to leave an adequately vascularised bed for a split skin graft to cover the flap donor site.

Flaps should not be based on the fallacious length:width ratio (8), but instead should be based on rational design to incorporate no more than one adjacent perforator (Figure 8.2). Distally based fasciocutaneous flaps are based on relatively constant septocutaneous perforators that arise from the posterior tibial artery and venae commitans around 10 and 15 cm proximal to the tip of the medial malleolus (9) (see Figure 3.1, Chapter 3). Like the proximally based flaps, the anterior border of the flap coincides with the medial fasciotomy incision, 1.5 cm posterior to the medial subcutaneous border of the tibia in adults. Extensive degloving precludes the use of these local flaps due to damage to the

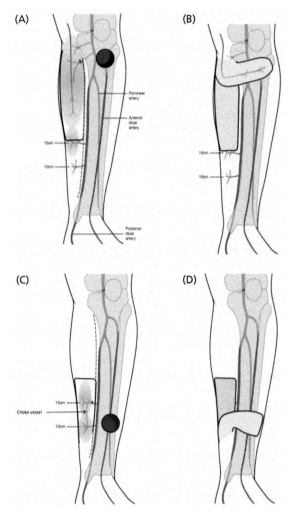

Figure 8.2 Local fasciocutaneous flap options. (a, b) Proximally based flap based on the medial inferior genicular artery/saphenous artery and proximally based perforators to cover defects around the knee. (c, d) Distally based flap based on the 10 cm perforator to cover distal third anterior tibial defects. Both flaps are planned so that the anterior border coincides with the medial fasciotomy incision. The donor site is then resurfaced with a split thickness skin graft.

perforators as well as the supra- and sub-fascial vascular plexuses. The dominant perforator is directly visualised and, if suitable, the flap is then planned in reverse to ensure that it can be transposed without undue tension. The long saphenous vein should either be excluded from the anterior border of the flap or, if this is not possible, ligated at the base of the flap to prevent venous congestion of the flap as the venae commitans of the perforator will struggle to cope with the venous drainage from the medial side of the foot. Like the proximally based flaps, the deep fascia is included to protect the prefascial vascular plexus. Islanding of the flaps to create the so-called propeller flaps allows turning through a greater angle and a neater inset but may be associated with increased complication rates. In a multicentre prospective study, the Lower Extremity Assessment Project (LEAP) Study Group found that use of local fasciocutaneous flaps for tibial defects following high-energy injuries was associated with higher complication rates compared with free flaps (10). Whilst there were no significant differences between the free and local flap groups with respect to overall complication rates, among those with the most severe grade of underlying bone injury, limbs treated with a local flap were 4.3 times more likely to have a wound complication requiring intervention than those treated with a free flap. In a systematic review and meta-analysis of 40 studies on perforator-pedicled propeller flaps in lower limb defects, of which 55.2% were post-traumatic, complications were found in 25.2%, with a partial necrosis rate of 10.2% and complete necrosis rate of 3.5% (11). The authors identified age of over 60 years, diabetes, and arteriopathy were significant risk factors.

The sural artery flap, based on the sural artery and venae commitans that accompany the sural nerve, has been advocated to cover defects in the lower third of the leg. The supplying perforator arises from the peroneal artery, which is often injured when the fibula fractures. A systematic review and pooled analysis of 907 patients with mixed indications including trauma (39.4%), ulcers (16.3%), and open fracture (10.5%) found a complication rate of 26.4%, with a total flap loss rate of 3.2% (12). However, a retrospective review of 70 sural artery flaps utilised for various indications including acute trauma reported an overall complication rate of 59%, with partial or tip or complete necrosis in 35% of all cases (13). Therefore, we do not recommend this flap for patients with open fractures.

Local muscle flaps

There are limited options for local muscle coverage in the lower limb (14). The medial or lateral heads of the gastrocnemius provide limited coverage around the knee but do not extend to cover the proximal pole of the patella or distally to the proximal third of tibia. The larger medial head can reach further and is therefore more commonly used. Whilst normal gait is possible following use of one head of the gasctronemius, functional deficit, including peak force generated during push-off, can be detected during more demanding tasks such as fast or uphill walking (15).

The soleus muscle flap has been used for coverage of middle third tibial defects if based proximally, or even distal third if based distally. However, in addition to the proximal pedicle, the muscle relies on multiple segmental perforators, some of which require division for mobilisation. This precarious blood supply together with its close proximity to the posterior surface of the tibia and inclusion in the zone of injury mean that it is an unreliable option for the reconstruction of open fractures (16).

A tibialis anterior muscle turnover flap can cover long narrow defects over the tibial crest but only for defects up to 1 cm wide (17).

Free flaps

Free tissue transfer has revolutionised the management of open fractures. Free flaps are preferred to local flap reconstruction for patients with multiple co-morbidities such as diabetes, venous insufficiency, and peripheral arterial disease. This subgroup of patients is at high risk of local flap failure and is often erroneously considered to be unsuitable for free flaps. Careful optimisation of the patient and techniques can result in free flap success rates in open fracture of over 90% and similar to those for elective reconstructive surgery (18). Microsurgical free tissue transfer also provides a wide choice for reconstruction of the defect. Flap selection depends on the size and location of the defect, location of the recipient vessels (which are ideally outside the zone of injury), as well as the biological contribution of the constituent tissues.

Fasciocutaneous versus muscle flaps

Every flap option is associated with its own advantages and disadvantages. Muscle flaps easily conform to complex defects. Although initially bulky, the oedema can be controlled with a pressure garment once the overlying skin graft is stable and any external fixator has been removed, and the denervated muscle soon atrophies and does not require thinning. A disadvantage of muscle flaps is that the overlying skin graft may be susceptible to minor trauma especially around the foot and ankle, and the flap can be difficult to raise and re-inset if further open surgery at the fracture site is required. Fasciocutaneous flaps have the advantage of replacing 'like with like' without sacrificing muscle function. They can be debulked by liposuction and can therefore provide a good contour and are more resilient to shear forces than a split skin graft.

There is no clinical evidence currently to support the use of one form of soft tissue cover over another for open fractures of the lower limb. Published evidence consists almost entirely of descriptive, retrospective, underpowered observational case series (level IV evidence) with major discrepancies in outcomes measures, thus precluding any meaningful meta-analysis. Few of these studies have compared muscle flaps with fasciocutaneous flaps specifically and those that did were limited by a lack of statistical power and case heterogeneity. A retrospective review of muscle and fascial flaps, both local and free, in lower extremity trauma found that complications were related to the severity of injury rather than the type of soft tissue coverage (19). Another study comparing muscle and fasciocutaneous flaps found that donor site morbidity was similar in both groups at around 4% (20). Comparison of free muscle and fasciocutaneous flaps for lower extremity reconstruction found no difference in major or minor complication rates (21), although patients who underwent fasciocutaneous flap reconstruction were more likely to require revision surgery to improve cosmesis. A retrospective review of patients with open tibial fractures treated with either free muscle or fasciocutaneous flaps showed that equivalent numbers went on to achieve bony union and could walk unaided by 2 years and there was no difference in the rates of complete flap survival and chronic osteomyelitis (22). The authors found that muscle conformed better to complex defects but fasciocutaneous flaps better tolerated secondary surgical procedures. Another recent retrospective review found similar rates of limb salvage and functional recovery when comparing muscle versus fasciocutaneous free flaps in acute traumatic injuries as well as chronic traumatic sequelae, with overall rates of flap loss and limb amputation of 8% and 6%, respectively (23). In patients with grade IIIB injuries and/or exposed defect hardware, fasciocutaneous flaps were more likely to require bone grafting for non-union compared with muscle flaps. It is not possible to determine whether this is due to differences in undocumented primary injury characteristics, the biological effect of the flap on bone repair, or other confounders.

In contrast, there is increasing experimental evidence to show that muscle coverage of diaphyseal fractures leads to superior fracture repair compared with fasciocutaneous tissue (24–28). Both fasciocutaneous and muscle flaps serve as a vascular supply to the fractured bone ends that have been stripped of periosteum and undergone disruption of the endosteum (24, 25, 28). Therefore, whilst vascularity is essential for fracture repair, other biological factors become limiting once the adequate blood supply threshold has been crossed. Although both fasciocutaneous tissue and muscle harbour mesenchymal stromal cells, human muscle-derived stromal cells exhibit significantly greater osteogenic potential than those from fasciocutaneous tissue, including both skin and adipose, and are equivalent to those from bone marrow (29). Therefore, muscle in direct apposition with diaphyseal fractures may promote repair by providing a readily available pool of mesenchymal stromal cells, which can undergo osteogenic differentiation into bone-forming osteoblasts especially in the post-traumatic inflammatory environment (29–31). Furthermore, muscle also provides an anabolic environment to bone through the expression of growth factors (32). Studies comparing bacterial clearance found superior elimination under muscle compared with fasciocutaneous tissue, despite a higher blood flow in the latter (33, 34).

In the absence of robust clinical evidence and based on the available experimental data, consideration may be given to the use of chimeric flaps, such as the free anterolateral thigh flap including a segment of vastus lateralis, to cover tibial shaft fractures (35). This would provide the advantage of avoiding the unsightly skin grafted donor site below the knee whilst retaining the biological benefits of muscle in direct apposition to the fracture site.

Recipient vessels for microsurgical anastomoses

The site of anastomoses to the recipient vessels should be selected ideally outside the zone of injury and preferably proximal to the defect. Intimal injury can be difficult to recognise from external inspection and anastomoses just proximal to a patent small vessel supplying the adjacent muscle ensures that the surgeon is outside the zone of injury. The posterior tibial vessels are less likely to have been injured during the initial trauma (36, 37) and are more reliable and accessible as recipient vessels than the anterior tibial vessels. In a retrospective review of 68 patients with open tibial fractures requiring free tissue transfer, 18 patients had 22 vascular injuries (4 patients had injuries to 2 vessels) that were diagnosed using pre-operative computed tomography (CT) angiography (38). In another series of severe open tibial injuries (37), 80.6% of 191 patients underwent vascular imaging. A total of 57.1% had abnormal findings on imaging compared with 11% on initial evaluation and there was a false positive rate of 7.8%. In a randomised controlled trial in 157 patients with isolated open tibial fractures and initially adequate circulation (39), the authors compared the outcomes of patients who underwent conventional wound excision and primary skeletal stabilisation with those who had routine exploration and repair of the major vessels and nerves. In the second group, 28.2% of patients were found to have occult major vascular injuries, and outcomes at both intermediate and long-term follow-up were superior. These studies suggest that preoperative vascular imaging can assist in preoperative planning. However, imaging of the vasculature should not delay operative intervention particularly when there is the limb is devascularised (see Chapter 10). In the UK, many emergency units now offer full body CT scans for trauma patients, hence CT angiogram should not cause excessive delays and is recommended.

We recommend that the artery is anastomosed end-to-side to preserve the distal vascular supply and a single vessel leg is not a contraindication to it being used as a recipient. At an incidence of 7.2%, venous insufficiency was the commonest cause of re-exploration in free tissue transfers to the lower extremity, and anastomoses to the superficial venous system group were associated with a higher rate of venous insufficiency and partial flap loss compared with the deep venous system group (40). The number of venous anastomoses that should be performed remains controversial. In elective free tissue transfer, the use of two venous anastomoses has been found to result in a significant reduction in the rate of venous congestion without significantly impacting on either complication rate or operative time (41). Two retrospective reviews of over 300 free flaps each for lower limb reconstruction found that anastomosis of one rather than two veins did not significantly reduce the rate of surgical complications including total flap loss (40, 42). However, a recent retrospective study of 361 free flaps for Gustilo–Anderson grade IIIB and IIIC injuries (43) found that two venous anastomoses demonstrated a four-fold decrease in complication rates compared with a single venous anastomosis. Furthermore, venous size mismatch of over 1 mm (when anastomosing large to small) was an independent predictive factor for total flap failure.

Many patients suffer from postoperative oedema of the lower limb and the flap. Various dangling protocols and compression stockings have been advocated to aid lymphatic and venous drainage. A recent systematic review of dangling regimes after free flap surgery to the lower limb (44) found that a 3-day flap training regime is sufficient for physiological training and that it may be appropriate to start dangling as early as postoperative day 3. However, robust evidence for dangling and compression is currently lacking (45, 46).

Conclusion

Definitive soft tissue coverage for open fractures should be achieved within 72 hours of the injury if it cannot be performed at the time of wound excision (47). If internal fixation is used, definitive coverage should be achieved at the same time (47). An understanding of the topography of angiosomes of the leg permits raising of local fasciocutaneous flaps reliably; these should be reserved for low-energy injuries where the flap donor site has not been degloved and, in the case of distally based flaps, direct visual inspection of the supplying perforator confirms suitability. High-energy fractures with a wide zone of injury suitable for reconstruction are best covered with free flaps, with the posterior tibial vessels as the preferred recipient vessels for defects over the leg.

References

1. **Chan JK, Harry L, Williams G, Nanchahal J.** Soft-tissue reconstruction of open fractures of the lower limb: muscle versus fasciocutaneous flaps. Plast Reconstr Surg. 2012;**130**(2):284e–95e.

2. **Hallock GG.** A paradigm shift in flap selection protocols for zones of the lower extremity using perforator flaps. J Reconstr Microsurg. 2013;**29**(4):233–40.

3. **Tajsic N, Winkel R, Husum H.** Distally based perforator flaps for reconstruction of post-traumatic defects of the lower leg and foot. A review of the anatomy and clinical outcomes. Injury. 2014;**45**(3):469–77.

4. **Whetzel TP, Barnard MA, Stokes RB.** Arterial fasciocutaneous vascular territories of the lower leg. Plast Reconstr Surg. 1997;**100**(5):1172–83; discussion 1184–5.

5. **Stadler F, Brenner E, Todoroff B, Papp C.** Anatomical study of the perforating vessels of the lower leg. Anat Rec. 1999;**255**(4):374–9.

6. **Drimouras G, Kostopoulos E, Agiannidis C, Papadodima S, Champsas G, Papoutsis I,** et al. Redefining vascular anatomy of posterior tibial artery perforators: a cadaveric study and review of the literature. Ann Plast Surg. 2016;**76**(6):705–12.

7. **Ghali S, Bowman N, Khan U.** The distal medial perforators of the lower leg and their accompanying veins. Br J Plast Surg. 2005;**58**(8):1086–9.

8. **Milton SH.** Pedicled skin-flaps: the fallacy of the length: width ratio. Br J Surg. 1970;**57**(7):502–8.

9. **Schaverien M, Saint-Cyr M.** Perforators of the lower leg: analysis of perforator locations and clinical application for pedicled perforator flaps. Plast Reconstr Surg. 2008;**122**(1):161–70.

10. **Pollak AN, McCarthy ML, Burgess AR.** Short-term wound complications after application of flaps for coverage of traumatic soft-tissue defects about the tibia. The Lower Extremity Assessment Project (LEAP) Study Group. J Bone Joint Surg Am. 2000;**82**-A(12):1681–91.

11. **Bekara F, Herlin C, Mojallal A, Sinna R, Ayestaray B, Letois F,** et al. A systematic review and meta-analysis of perforator-pedicled propeller flaps in lower extremity defects: identification of risk factors for complications. Plast Reconstr Surg. 2016;**137**(1):314–31.

12. **de Blacam C, Colakoglu S, Ogunleye AA, Nguyen JT, Ibrahim AM, Lin SJ,** et al. Risk factors associated with complications in lower-extremity reconstruction with the distally based sural flap: a systematic review and pooled analysis. J Plast Reconstr Aesthet Surg. 2014;**67**(5):607–16.

13. **Baumeister SP, Spierer R, Erdmann D, Sweis R, Levin LS, Germann GK.** A realistic complication analysis of 70 sural artery flaps in a multimorbid patient group. Plast Reconstr Surg. 2003;**112**(1):129–40; discussion 141–2.

14. **d'Avila F, Franco D, d'Avila B, Arnaut M, Jr.** Use of local muscle flaps to cover leg bone exposures. Rev Col Bras Cir. 2014;**41**(6):434–9.

15. **Kramers-de Quervain IA, Lauffer JM, Kach K, Trentz O, Stussi E.** Functional donor-site morbidity during level and uphill gait after a gastrocnemius or soleus muscle-flap procedure. J Bone Joint Surg Am. 2001;**83**-A(2):239–46.

16. **Tobin GR.** Soleus flaps. In: **Strauch BV, Hall-Findlay, E, Lee, B,** eds. Grabb's Encyclopedia of Flaps. 3rd ed. Philadelphia, PA: Wolters Kluwer, Lippincott Williams & Wilkins; 2009. pp. 1394–8.

17. **Pers MM, S.; Kirkby, B.** Tibialis anterior muscle flap. In: **Strauch BV, Hall-Findlay, E, Lee, B,** eds. Grabb's Encyclopedia of Flaps. 3rd ed. Philadelphia, PA: Wolters Kluwer, Lippincott Williams & Wilkins; 2009. pp. 1398–400.

18. **Gardiner MD, Nanchahal J.** Strategies to ensure success of microvascular free tissue transfer. J Plast Reconstr Aesthet Surg. 2010;**63**(9):e665–73.

19. **Hallock GG.** Utility of both muscle and fascia flaps in severe lower extremity trauma. J Trauma. 2000;**48**(5):913–17.

20. **Hallock GG.** Relative donor-site morbidity of muscle and fascial flaps. Plast Reconstr Surg. 1993;**92**(1):70–6.

21. **Paro J, Chiou G, Sen SK.** Comparing muscle and fasciocutaneous free flaps in lower extremity reconstruction—does it matter? Ann Plast Surg. 2016;**76**(Suppl 3):S213–15.

22. **Yazar S, Lin CH, Lin YT, Ulusal AE, Wei FC.** Outcome comparison between free muscle and free fasciocutaneous flaps for reconstruction of distal third and ankle traumatic open tibial fractures. Plast Reconstr Surg. 2006;**117**(7):2468–75; discussion 2476–7.

23. **Cho EH, Shammas RL, Carney MJ, Weissler JM, Bauder AR, Glener AD,** et al. Muscle versus fasciocutaneous free flaps in lower extremity traumatic reconstruction: a multicenter outcomes analysis. Plast Reconstr Surg. 2018;**141**(1):191–9.

24. **Harry LE, Sandison A, Paleolog EM, Hansen U, Pearse MF, Nanchahal J.** Comparison of the healing of open tibial fractures covered with either muscle or fasciocutaneous tissue in a murine model. J Orthop Res. 2008;**26**(9):1238–44.

25. **Harry LE, Sandison A, Pearse MF, Paleolog EM, Nanchahal J.** Comparison of the vascularity of fasciocutaneous tissue and muscle for coverage of open tibial fractures. Plast Reconstr Surg. 2009;**124**(4):1211–9.

26. **Richards RR, McKee MD, Paitich CB, Anderson GI, Bertoia JT.** A comparison of the effects of skin coverage and muscle flap coverage on the early strength of union at the site of osteotomy after devascularization of a segment of canine tibia. J Bone Joint Surg Am. 1991;**73**(9):1323–30.

27. **Richards RR, Orsini EC, Mahoney JL, Verschuren R.** The influence of muscle flap coverage on the repair of devascularized tibial cortex: an experimental investigation in the dog. Plast Reconstr Surg. 1987;**79**(6):946–58.

28. **Richards RR, Schemitsch EH.** Effect of muscle flap coverage on bone blood flow following devascularization of a segment of tibia: an experimental investigation in the dog. J Orthop Res. 1989;**7**(4):550–8.

29. **Glass GE, Chan JK, Freidin A, Feldmann M, Horwood NJ, Nanchahal J.** TNF-alpha promotes fracture repair by augmenting the recruitment and differentiation of muscle-derived stromal cells. Proc Natl Acad Sci U S A. 2011;**108**(4):1585–90.

30. **Dey D, Bagarova J, Hatsell SJ, Armstrong KA, Huang L, Ermann J,** et al. Two tissue-resident progenitor lineages drive distinct phenotypes of heterotopic ossification. Sci Transl Med. 2016;**8**(366):366ra163.

31. **Chan JK, Glass GE, Ersek A, Freidin A, Williams GA, Gowers K,** et al. Low-dose TNF augments fracture healing in normal and osteoporotic bone by up-regulating the innate immune response. EMBO Mol Med. 2015;**7**(5):547–61.

32. **Pedersen BK.** Muscles and their myokines. J Exp Biol. 2011;**214**(Pt 2):337–46.

33. **Calderon W, Chang N, Mathes SJ.** Comparison of the effect of bacterial inoculation in musculocutaneous and fasciocutaneous flaps. Plast Reconstr Surg. 1986;**77**(5):785–94.

34. **Gosain A, Chang N, Mathes S, Hunt TK, Vasconez L.** A study of the relationship between blood flow and bacterial inoculation in musculocutaneous and fasciocutaneous flaps. Plast Reconstr Surg. 1990;**86**(6):1152–62; discussion 1163.

35. **Zheng X, Zheng C, Wang B, Qiu Y, Zhang Z, Li H, et al.** Reconstruction of complex soft-tissue defects in the extremities with chimeric anterolateral thigh perforator flap. Int J Surg. 2016;**26**:25–31.

36. **Chen HC, Chuang CC, Chen S, Hsu WM, Wei FC.** Selection of recipient vessels for free flaps to the distal leg and foot following trauma. Microsurgery. 1994;**15**(5):358–63.

37. **Haddock NT, Weichman KE, Reformat DD, Kligman BE, Levine JP, Saadeh PB.** Lower extremity arterial injury patterns and reconstructive outcomes in patients with severe lower extremity trauma: a 26-year review. J Am Coll Surg. 2010;**210**(1):66–72.

38. **Chummun S, Wigglesworth TA, Young K, Healey B, Wright TC, Chapman TW, et al.** Does vascular injury affect the outcome of open tibial fractures? Plast Reconstr Surg. 2013;**131**(2):303–9.

39. **Waikakul S, Sakkarnkosol S, Vanadurongwan V.** Vascular injuries in compound fractures of the leg with initially adequate circulation. J Bone Joint Surg Br. 1998;**80**(2):254–8.

40. **Lorenzo AR, Lin CH, Lin CH, Lin YT, Nguyen A, Hsu CC, et al.** Selection of the recipient vein in microvascular flap reconstruction of the lower extremity: analysis of 362 free-tissue transfers. J Plast Reconstr Aesthet Surg. 2011;**64**(5):649–55.

41. **Enajat M, Rozen WM, Whitaker IS, Smit JM, Acosta R.** A single center comparison of one versus two venous anastomoses in 564 consecutive DIEP flaps: investigating the effect on venous congestion and flap survival. Microsurgery. 2010;**30**(3):185–91.

42. **Heidekrueger PI, Ehrl D, Heine-Geldern A, Ninkovic M, Broer PN.** One versus two venous anastomoses in microvascular lower extremity reconstruction using gracilis muscle or anterolateral thigh flaps. Injury. 2016;**47**(12):2828–32.

43. **Stranix JT, Lee ZH, Anzai L, Jacoby A, Avraham T, Saadeh PB, et al.** Optimizing venous outflow in reconstruction of Gustilo IIIB lower extremity traumas with soft tissue free flap coverage: are two veins better than one? Microsurgery. 2017;**38**(7):745–51.

44. **McGhee JT, Cooper L, Orkar K, Harry L, Cubison T.** Systematic review: early versus late dangling after free flap reconstruction of the lower limb. J Plast Reconstr Aesthet Surg. 2017;**70**(8):1017–27.

45. **Cerny M, Schantz JT, Erne H, Schmauss D, Giunta RE, Machens HG, et al.** [Overview and introduction of a treatment concept for postoperative care and mobilisation after free flap transplantation in the lower extremity]. Handchir Mikrochir Plast Chir. 2016;**48**(6):363–9.

46. **Rohde C, Howell BW, Buncke GM, Gurtner GC, Levin LS, Pu LL, et al.** A recommended protocol for the immediate postoperative care of lower extremity free-flap reconstructions. J Reconstr Microsurg. 2009;**25**(1):15–9.

47. **National Institute for Health and Care Excellence (NICE).** NICE guidance: fractures (complex). 2016. https://www.nice.org.uk/guidance/ng37/evidence

Chapter 9

Bone Loss in Open Fractures

Summary

1. Bone loss in relation to open fractures may arise directly from extrusion of fragments at the time of injury or after surgical excision (debridement).
2. Safe and effective management requires expertise of both plastic and orthopaedic specialists in reconstruction. These cases are particularly challenging and should be managed in units with relevant expertise and experience.
3. The options for reconstruction will depend on the shape and size of the defect, the location within the bone, the condition of the local soft tissue, and the patient's general physical and mental health.
4. Bone defects can be reconstructed through autogenous bone grafts (with or without augmentation), vascularised free transfer of bone (usually the fibula), or by distraction osteogenesis (according to the methods described by Ilizarov).

Introduction

This chapter deals with the management of bone loss in open fractures with particular reference to the tibia. This is a challenging problem and requires input and expertise from orthopaedic and plastic surgery specialists in limb reconstruction. The different sizes, shapes, and location of the defect will have diverse implications and management must be individualised.

Aetiology of bone loss

Bone loss can occur from the initial injury (extrusion of bone fragments or segments at the time of impact) or following wound excision in open fractures. High-energy trauma to the metaphysis of osteoporotic bone can lead to crushing with impaction of cancellous bone that, in effect, creates a defect even without there being any physical removal of bone. Pathological fractures, too, may present with bone loss consequent to both the pathological process and the injury.

Types of defect

Cavitary or contained

This type of defect is a closed cavity seen after impaction in cancellous bone of the metaphysis of long bones or in the calcaneum.

Partial

Partial defects occur when a proportion of the circumference of a bone has been lost. Amenable to replacement by bone grafting when small, these are more challenging if involving an articular surface. After wound excision if most of the circumference has been lost, the surgeon may choose to create a true segmental defect in order to facilitate techniques such as bone transport.

True segmental

Segmental defects are created when the full circumference of bone over a length is lost. This occurs typically in the diaphysis of long bones.

Modes of treatment

Expectant or non-surgical (conservative)

Spontaneous restoration may be seen in young children, usually under the age of 6 years. In adults this phenomenon is observed occasionally in those patients who have had significant head trauma associated with the limb injuries. This pattern of spontaneous replacement happens more frequently in the femur than the tibia. The key in any expectant approach is a serial evaluation of clinical and radiological signs. The absence of continued progress should prompt intervention.

Bone grafting

Autogenous bone graft remains a benchmark for treating bone defects against which other methods are compared. It is used for defects from open fractures after satisfactory wound healing; use at the time of index wound excision or before definitive wound healing may potentially increase the risk of infection through the introduction of non-vascularised material into a contaminated bed. Bone grafting procedures carry some donor site morbidity and have limitations in terms of volume and biological activity (particularly in older patients and those with immune suppression). Consequently, different methods of augmenting the volume and activity of autogenous bone graft have been proposed:

Induced membrane technique

The induced membrane by Masquelet is a method for augmenting bone grafting procedures (1). An antibiotic-loaded polymethylmethacrylate (PMMA) cement spacer is placed and moulded to cover the bone at both ends of the defect at the time of soft tissue cover or wound closure. This induces a foreign body reaction producing a biologically active membrane around it that is highly vascular and has cells producing osteogenic growth factors. The cement spacer maintains the length of the limb, provides effective dead space management, and delivers a high concentration of antibiotics locally. The technique is illustrated in Figure 9.1.

Maturation of the membrane (from 6–12 weeks) is followed by a second procedure to remove the cement spacer and replace this with autogenous bone graft. The membrane is incised and protected when the cement spacer is extracted so that closure will facilitate containment of the graft material within the defect. The bone edges at either end of the defect are inspected, excised further if needed, and sharply 'petalled' (osteoperiosteal and cortical leaves are elevated from the surface of bone to stimulate a new inflammatory response) before the graft is placed.

Bone graft is obtained from the iliac crest or femoral canal (using the RIA—reamer irrigator aspirator—technique) as large volumes may be required (2, 3). Whilst the induced membrane technique is itself an augmentation procedure for autogenous bone graft, some parties advocate addition of further adjuncts such as bone morphogenetic proteins or bone marrow aspirate-concentrated osteoprogenitor cells.

Good results have been reported using this technique, particularly in the upper limb and femur (1, 4). In the tibia, Masquelet has encouraged creating cross-unions between the tibia and fibula at levels proximal to and distal to the level of the defect especially when external fixation is utilised for stabilisation. This is said to reduce refractures after fixator removal.

The induced membrane technique, especially when used in combination with internal fixation, may be more acceptable than prolonged external fixation and bone transport. It is helpful for partial or oblique defects where, if bone transport were performed, docking of bone ends might be troublesome. However, complications do occur and some centres have reported less favourable results in the tibia (5).

Where complex plastic surgery has been performed for definitive wound cover, and the induced membrane technique is considered, some pre-emptive discussions with plastic surgical colleagues will help in planning for access through this cover for bone grafting.

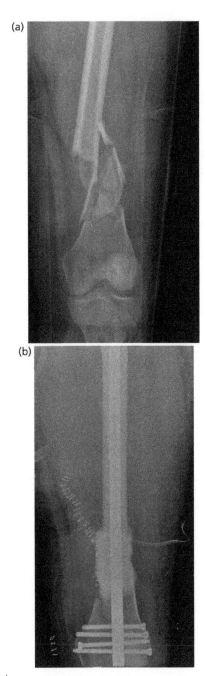

Figure 9.1 Continued

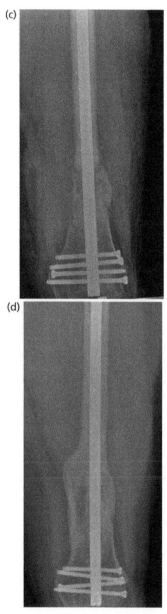

Figure 9.1 Radiographs showing the induced membrane technique (Masquelet) used to treat a segmental bone defect after an open fracture of the femur. There was a large antero-medial wound (a). At wound excision, a large volume of distal diaphyseal bone, found to be completely devitalised, was removed producing a 10 cm segmental defect. A locked retrograde femoral nail was used to stabilise the fracture, a polymethylmethacrylate cement spacer placed in the bone defect and the wound closed primarily (b). Ten weeks post-injury, the cement spacer was removed and reamer irrigator aspirator harvested bone graft inserted into the membrane (c). The graft was fully incorporated at 18 months (d).

Bone graft substitutes

These are natural, synthetic, and animal-derived osteoconductive scaffolds and are available in many forms including structural blocks, chips, pellets, granules, and injectable cements (6). Some have been employed effectively for contained periarticular defects in closed fractures but using inert material in open fractures where the surgical field may, despite the best excision and lavage, still hold elements of contamination increases the risk of deep infection.

Bone graft substitutes can serve as a volume expander when using autogenous bone graft in the Masquelet method; the field is unlikely to be contaminated owing to the period of exposure to local antibiotics and the observation of satisfactory wound healing (1, 4).

Bone graft adjuncts

Various commercially available products have been developed to act as biological response modifiers to bone healing. Whilst some have been used in isolation for other indications, it is more usual to combine these with autogenous bone grafts when managing critical-sized segmental defects. Examples include the bone morphogenic proteins (BMPs), bone marrow and blood derivatives, and demineralised bone matrix.

BMPs are signalling proteins in the recruitment of osteoprogenitor cells during fracture healing. Originally described by Urist (7), commercial preparations of recombinant BMP-2 promoted fracture healing and bony union (8, 9) including in open tibial fractures (10, 11). The Food and Drug Administration (FDA) in the US thus approved BMP use in the treatment of acute tibial fractures managed with intramedullary fixation (12). However, recent studies have failed to find conclusive evidence for clinical effectiveness (13, 14); calls for adequately powered randomised trials to validate its continued use have occurred (12).

Bone marrow aspirate concentrate (BMAC) enables a harvest and concentrate of mesenchymal stem cells (MSCs), usually from iliac crest bone marrow, for clinical application. Laboratory studies suggest that MSCs can provide both a source of bone-healing cells and relevant cellular signalling molecules (15), with some clinical studies suggesting a use in augmenting bone healing during distraction osteogenesis and bone grafting procedures (15).

Platelet-rich plasma (PRP) is a blood derivative obtained by centrifugation of the patient's blood. It contains very high concentrations of growth factors relevant to bone healing but preclinical work assessing the effectiveness of PRP in bone healing is limited. Whilst both BMAC and PRP procedures appear safe and research activity into potential clinical application is ongoing, specific recommendation for use in open fractures is premature (15, 16).

Demineralised bone graft is allogenic bone processed to remove mineral and cellular components. It contains bone matrix proteins and osteo-inductive cellular signalling molecules including BMPs. Although some studies describe its use as a bone graft substitute and expander, clinical evidence for effectiveness is weak and no studies for a role in open fracture defects exist. It is thus not recommended at the current time (17).

Vascularised bone grafting

The fibula, with its peroneal artery pedicle and hence vascular supply intact, is the most common bone transferred for tibial bone defects. It can be transferred ipsilaterally through a proximal and distal osteotomy and the intermediate segment slowly moved across from posterolateral to anteromedial to bridge the gap created from a tibial defect (18). This technique of slow transfer is achieved usually in an Ilizarov fixator and is termed transverse bone transport to distinguish it from longitudinal bone transport (described in further detail later in the chapter). The gradual transfer preserves the vascularity of the fibula segment. Alternatively, the fibula can be transferred as a vascularised graft from the contralateral leg; microsurgical anastomosis of the peroneal artery of the fibula to a suitable vascular bundle in the host (recipient) leg is required to re-establish the blood supply (19). An example of a free fibula microvascular transfer is shown in Figure 9.2.

This form of bone replacement for tibial defects carries the advantage of long defects being adequately filled by a corresponding length of fibula. It is also suited for partial defects of the tibia in which a small circumference of the tibia remains but over a long length; the fibula can be inserted and fixed to the remaining circumference thereby avoiding conversion of the defect into a segmental type by excising the remaining viable part (Figure 9.2).

This method of replacement requires the expertise of either a surgeon trained in transverse bone transport or one in free vascularised bone transfer. In the latter, considerations should be made for the impact of loss of the fibula from the contralateral leg (there can be restrictions on sports activities and problems with a deformity of the great toe) and the period of protection and activity modification required (usually 18 months or longer) until the transferred fibula has hypertrophied and is capable of load transfer equivalent to the intact tibia.

Distraction osteogenesis (DO)

DO is the most established method of bone regeneration for large segment bone loss (20). The technique employs the 'tension stress effect' whereby gradual traction on biological tissues induces metabolic activity, cellular proliferation and tissue synthesis (21). The technique has found multiple applications in

(a)

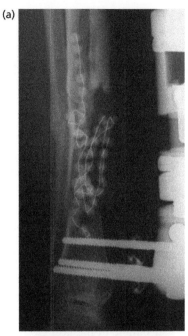

(b)

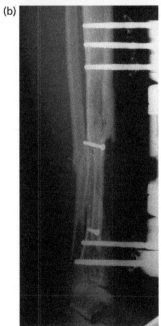

Figure 9.2 Continued

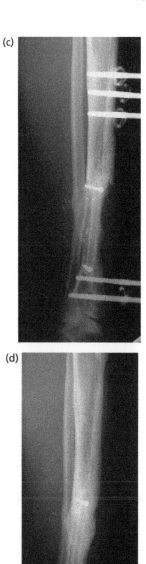

Figure 9.2 Clinical photographs and radiographs showing the use of a free fibula to treat an open fracture of the tibia with a long partial defect. After wound excision gentamicin beads were used to manage the dead space (a). This was then replaced by a vascularised free fibula transfer that was internally fixed with screws and the entire tibia supported by a spanning external fixator until union (b and c). It took approximately 18 months for the fibula to hypertrophy (d).

orthopaedic surgery for bone regeneration in various situations (22). An example of bone restoration by distraction osteogenesis is shown in Figure 9.3.

DO is carried out usually with a circular (Ilizarov) external fixator. A stable arrangement of rings is applied and a low-energy corticotomy (technique of osteotomy) undertaken. This is followed by a **latent phase** of usually 7–14 days which allows for the formation of early repair tissue that is biologically active and that will respond favourably to mechanical stimulus. During the subsequent **distraction phase**, traction is applied usually at a rate of 0.25 mm four times a day (1 mm in total). This rate of distraction has been associated with the most reliable bone formation. Once the desired length has been achieved it is necessary to hold the bone segment in position with sufficient stability to allow the newly formed bone to consolidate. The external fixator is maintained **in situ** (or replaced with alternative forms of internal stabilisation) during this **consolidation phase**; the average total time in the external fixator is between 1 and 2 months per centimetre of bone regeneration.

The ability to solve the problem of bone defects by a percutaneous technique and external fixation, and avoid the use of internal implants in an at-risk environment for infection, is particularly attractive in open fractures (20). This must be balanced against the incumbency of prolonged external fixation and the potential for adverse events such as pin-site infections, joint contractures, and fixation failure.

Modifications to the standard technique of DO are used in order to improve patient experience and outcome whilst reducing complications. These include multifocal transport (using multiple distraction sites), acute shortening across the bone defect and lengthening from a distant site in the same bone, and combining the technique with internal fixation (20). Intramedullary devices that allow distraction osteogenesis without the need for external fixation have also been developed (23). There is insufficient evidence currently for specific recommendations using these modified techniques for bone defects in open fractures.

Bone loss in open tibial fractures—recommendations for management

Cavitary or contained (metaphyseal areas)

If the area of loss is small or unlikely to compromise support of the subarticular scaffold then an expectant approach is justified. If the area is large or replacement needed in the metaphyseal area to maintain articular stability or reinforce fixation, autogenous bone graft is used. Bone graft substitutes have been used successfully in this situation for closed periarticular fractures. Caution is

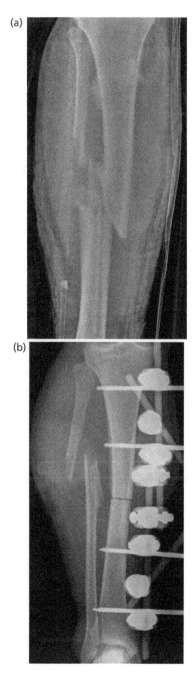

Figure 9.3 Continued

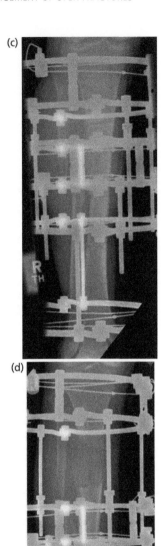

Figure 9.3 Continued

(e)

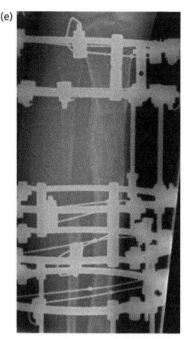

Figure 9.3 Radiographs and clinical photographs illustrating the use of distraction osteogenesis for acute bone loss after a high-energy open fracture of the tibia (a). Excision of devitalised bone and acute shortening across the defect allowed direct closure of the wound over bone and skin grafting of exposed muscle (b). The Ilizarov fixator has been applied and a proximal metaphyseal corticotomy performed (c). Lengthening has been completed and regenerate bone is visible in the distraction gap early (d) and late (e) in the reconstruction.

advised against use of this in open fractures; if used, the clinical indications would follow those as suggested for the use of internal fixation in open tibial injuries.

Partial defects

Small

This describes an area of subcritical bone loss judged unlikely to compromise union, usually less than 25% the circumference of the tibia. Complete healing will depend not only on the size but the geometry, location, and patient factors (including age and co-morbidities) that may affect union and stability. An expectant approach can be taken initially and if there is failure to progress after serial observations, autogenous bone graft is used.

Large

Critically sized defects are those felt likely to compromise union either from their location and influence on stability or through the lack of bone contact. There is a greater than 50% chance that additional procedures are required to accomplish fracture union if the defect is greater than 1 cm and the circumferential loss greater than 50% (24). The method of dealing with such a defect in an open tibial fracture can be through:

1. The induced membrane technique (see previous description).
2. Converting the partial defect to a complete segmental void and to reconstruct using distraction osteogenesis.
3. Vascularised bone graft (fibula).
4. Partial segment bone transport (hemi-callotasis).

Hemi-callotasis is a variant of bone transport but here, instead of a complete segment of bone that is gradually moved across a defect, a large fragment from division of part of the cortex of the tibia (usually the anterior circumference) is transported gradually across the defect, leaving a trail of new bone in its wake (Figure 6.4).

Segmental defects

Small (<3 cm)

Defects less than 15 mm may be left to heal by obliterating the defect through shortening the limb to facilitate contact between the bone ends and subsequent union. Some patients are better suited to achieving early fracture union without resorting to reconstruction of the bone defect as this may prolong the treatment period and recovery. The shortened limb may then be managed by orthotic means or not at all if less than 15 mm. However, larger defects towards 3 cm may be amenable to management by bone grafting after the soft tissues have recovered well or through use of the Masquelet technique as a planned procedure.

Large (>3 cm)

1. Distraction osteogenesis through segmental bone transport (see previously).
2. Acute closure of the defect by shortening and restoration of length by distraction osteogenesis.
3. Vascularised bone graft (fibula—ipsilateral or contralateral).
4. Induced membrane technique.

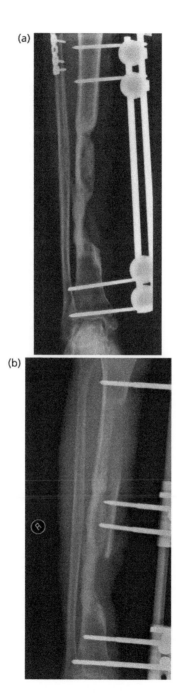

Figure 9.4 Continued

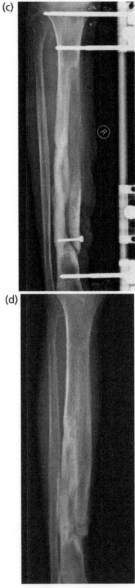

Figure 9.4 Radiographs showing a partial defect of the tibia (a) managed by the technique of bone transport of a fragment of cortical wall across the defect (hemi-callotasis). A portion of the cortical wall is osteotomised and held by external fixator pins. This is then gradually moved across the defect, leaving a trail of new bone in its wake (b). After docking of the portion of bone distally, internal fixation is added to assist fragment contact and union (c, d). (Images courtesy of Professor Huang Lei, Beijing Ji Shui Tan Hospital)

Conclusion

The management of bone defects from open tibial trauma requires the expertise of orthopaedic and plastic surgeons trained in reconstruction. There are a variety of techniques available to solve the problem. Individualisation of treatment entails an assessment of the local, systemic, and patient-related factors such that the optimum mode of treatment is chosen.

References

1. Masquelet AC, Begue T. The concept of induced membrane for reconstruction of long bone defects. Orthop Clinics. 2010;41(1):27–37.
2. Dawson J, Kiner D, Gardner WI, Swafford R, Nowotarski PJ. The reamer–irrigator–aspirator as a device for harvesting bone graft compared with iliac crest bone graft: union rates and complications. J Orthop Trauma. 2014;28(10):584–90.
3. Haubruck P, Ober J, Heller R, Miska M, Schmidmaier G, Tanner MC. Complications and risk management in the use of the reaming-irrigator-aspirator (RIA) system: RIA is a safe and reliable method in harvesting autologous bone graft. PLoS ONE. 2018;13(4):e0196051.
4. Giannoudis PV, Harwood PJ, Tosounidis T, Kanakaris NK. Restoration of long bone defects treated with the induced membrane technique: protocol and outcomes. Injury. 2016;47(Suppl 6):S53–S61.
5. Morris R, Hossain M, Evans A, Pallister I. Induced membrane technique for treating tibial defects gives mixed results. Bone Joint J. 2017;99-B(5):680–5.
6. Campana V, Milano G, Pagano E, Barba M, Cicione C, Salonna G, et al. Bone substitutes in orthopaedic surgery: from basic science to clinical practice. J Mat Sci Mat Med. 2014;25(10):2445–61.
7. Urist MR, Strates BS. Bone morphogenetic protein. J Dent Res. 1971;50(6):1392–406.
8. Dai J, Li L, Jiang C, Wang C, Chen H, Chai Y. Bone morphogenetic protein for the healing of tibial fracture: a meta-analysis of randomized controlled trials. PLoS ONE. 2015;10(10):e0141670.
9. Hagen A, Gorenoi V, Schonermark MP. Bone graft substitutes for the treatment of traumatic fractures of the extremities. GMS Health Technol Assess. 2012;8:Doc04.
10. Govender S, Csimma C, Genant HK, Valentin-Opran A, Amit Y, Arbel R, et al. Recombinant human bone morphogenetic protein-2 for treatment of open tibial fractures: a prospective, controlled, randomized study of four hundred and fifty patients. J Bone Joint Surg Am. 2002;84-A(12):2123–34.
11. Wei S, Cai X, Huang J, Xu F, Liu X, Wang Q. Recombinant human BMP-2 for the treatment of open tibial fractures. Orthopedics. 2012;35(6):e847–54.
12. Argintar E, Edwards S, Delahay J. Bone morphogenetic proteins in orthopaedic trauma surgery. Injury. 2011;42(8):730–4.
13. Garrison KR, Shemilt I, Donell S, Ryder JJ, Mugford M, Harvey I, et al. Bone morphogenetic protein (BMP) for fracture healing in adults. Cochrane Database Syst Rev. 2010(6):CD006950.

14. Lyon T, Scheele W, Bhandari M, Koval KJ, Sanchez EG, Christensen J, et al. Efficacy and safety of recombinant human bone morphogenetic protein-2/calcium phosphate matrix for closed tibial diaphyseal fracture: a double-blind, randomized, controlled phase-II/III trial. J Bone Joint Surg Am. 2013;**95**(23):2088–96.

15. Imam MA, Holton J, Ernstbrunner L, Pepke W, Grubhofer F, Narvani A, et al. A systematic review of the clinical applications and complications of bone marrow aspirate concentrate in management of bone defects and nonunions. Int Orthop. 2017;**41**(11):2213–20.

16. Roffi A, Di Matteo B, Krishnakumar GS, Kon E, Filardo G. Platelet-rich plasma for the treatment of bone defects: from pre-clinical rational to evidence in the clinical practice. A systematic review. Int Orthop. 2017;**41**(2):221–37.

17. van der Stok J, Hartholt KA, Schoenmakers DAL, Arts JJC. The available evidence on demineralised bone matrix in trauma and orthopaedic surgery: a systematic review. Bone Joint Res. 2017;**6**(7):423–32.

18. Meselhy MA, Singer MS, Halawa AM, Hosny GA, Adawy AH, Essawy OM. Gradual fibular transfer by Ilizarov external fixator in post-traumatic and post-infection large tibial bone defects. Arch Orthop Trauma Surg. 2018;**138**(5):653–60.

19. Sparks DS, Saleh DB, Rozen WM, Hutmacher DW, Schuetz MA, Wagels M. Vascularised bone transfer: history, blood supply and contemporary problems. J Plast, Reconstr Aesthet Surg. 2017;**70**(1):1–11.

20. Quinnan SM. Segmental bone loss reconstruction using ring fixation. J Orthop Trauma. 2017;**31** Suppl 5:S42–6.

21. Ilizarov GA. The Tension-Stress Effect on the Genesis and Growth of Tissues. Transosseous Osteosynthesis: Theoretical and Clinical Aspects of the Regeneration and Growth of Tissue. Berlin, Heidelberg, Germany: Springer Berlin Heidelberg; 1992. pp. 137–255.

22. Gubin A, Borzunov D, Malkova T. Ilizarov method for bone lengthening and defect management review of contemporary literature. Bull Hosp Jt Dis. 2016;**74**(2):145–54.

23. Rozbruch SR, Birch JG, Dahl MT, Herzenberg JE. Motorized intramedullary nail for management of limb-length discrepancy and deformity. JAAOS. 2014;**22**(7):403–9.

24. Sanders DW, Bhandari M, Guyatt G, Heels-Ansdell D, Schemitsch EH, Swiontkowski M, et al. Critical-sized defect in the tibia: is it critical? Results from the SPRINT trial. J Orthop Trauma. 2014;**28**(11):632–5.

Chapter 10

Vascular Injuries

Summary

1. Resuscitation and management of life-threatening injuries must take priority over any extremity problems.

2. Haemorrhage from the extremities must be controlled by direct pressure or tourniquet.

3. Use hard signs (lack of palpable pulses, continued blood loss, or expanding haematoma) to diagnose vascular injury. Do not rely on capillary return or Doppler signal to exclude vascular injury. The pink pulseless limb must be assumed to have an arterial injury until proven otherwise.

4. Devascularised limbs are a clinical emergency. If following fracture and joint reduction the limb remains devascularised, immediate surgical exploration is essential.

5. Revascularisation must take place as soon as possible and definitely within 3–4 hours as both muscle and neural tissue are especially susceptible to hypoxia.

6. Preoperative angiography is not necessary and wastes valuable time. The site of vascular injury can usually be ascertained from the mechanism of injury, fracture location and configuration, and by clinical examination. In a patient with multi-level trauma to the same limb or polytrauma who is undergoing a computed tomography (CT) scan, CT angiography may be helpful.

7. The use of vascular shunts revascularises the limb rapidly, minimising ischaemia time. Systemic anticoagulation is not necessary.

8. Once circulation is restored and an adequate reperfusion interval observed, re-evaluate the potential for limb salvage.

9. If salvage is deemed appropriate, perform skeletal fixation followed by definitive vascular repair followed by definitive soft tissue cover as required.

10. Access incisions for vascular repair must take into account the potential need for compartment decompression and definitive skeletal and soft tissue reconstruction.

11. Peripheral nerves that have been transected should be repaired immediately when possible. Crushed or contused nerves should be documented and followed up for evidence of recovery.

12. In patients with a single patent artery (usually posterior tibial) free flaps can be anastomosed end to side if required for soft tissue reconstruction.

Introduction

Open extremity fractures occur in an environment of high energy transfer. Consequently, systemic injuries should be suspected in all cases and emergency management approached in accordance with advanced trauma life support (ATLS) principles, recognising the primacy of airway management and cervical spine stabilisation, oxygenation and ventilation, and fluid resuscitation. Rarely, an open extremity fracture is associated with major haemorrhage. Importantly, control of catastrophic haemorrhage is now addressed at the first stage of the primary survey together with airway management and cervical spine stabilisation, CABCDE (Circulation (exsanguinating haemorrhage), Airway, Breathing, Circulation, Disability, Exposure). Major haemorrhage control may be achieved by applying direct pressure to the source of major bleeding, thereby maintaining such tissue perfusion as exists. In the field, the use of a tourniquet may save lives (1). If used, the time applied must be noted or written on the tourniquet to avoid unnecessarily prolonged ischaemia in the event of successful retrieval. Blind clamping of an actively bleeding vessel is potentially detrimental to vascular tissue and accompanying nerves and should be avoided (2).

Whether accompanied by major haemorrhage or not, a devascularised limb associated with an open fracture, designated 'IIIC' by the amended Gustilo–Anderson classification (3), is a clinical emergency requiring prompt recognition and treatment. Recognition is based on hard clinical signs, including lack of palpable pulses, continued bleeding, or an expanding haematoma (4). If possible, the quality of the pulses should be compared to the uninjured contralateral limb. Fractures or joint dislocations should be reduced as this may restore distal circulation. Pulses may be weak if the patient is hypovolaemic and this should be corrected. Assessment of pulses should not rely on the use of Doppler ultrasound and the ankle-brachial pressure index (ABPI) is associated with a substantial false negative rate (4) and inter-observer variability (5). Capillary refill time is a poor indicator of vascular compromise as pooling of blood in the limb may give the impression of slow capillary return.

The common injury patterns associated with loss of distal perfusion are:

1. Fracture of the femur with an associated wedge-shaped or butterfly fragment at a level close to Hunter's canal where the superficial femoral artery

comes closest to the posteromedial surface of the femur. These are often closed injuries.

2. Fracture dislocations of the knee.

3. Fracture dislocations of the ankle. The distal pulses often return following reduction of the dislocation and skeletal realignment.

4. Injury to all three vessels distal to the trifurcation. This vascular injury pattern is associated with severe soft tissue and bony injury; there is often non-viable muscle in multiple compartments and segmental bone loss. This patient group may be best served by expeditious amputation (Chapter 12).

Diagnosis

There are no randomised controlled trials linking diagnostic strategy with patient outcomes (4). Rather, the published data report the relative sensitivities and specificities of the various diagnostic strategies (CT angiography, Doppler ABPI <0.90) and clinical examination to a control (usually invasive angiography). In this instance sensitivity is more important than specificity as the consequences of a false negative are likely to be more severe than those of a false positive (unnecessary intervention). Whilst CT angiography exhibited 100% sensitivity and specificity, an error of interpretation was noted in two cases. Importantly, the time required for an additional visit to the CT suite for angiography was considered to add an unacceptable delay. However, many patients with open fractures will have an early trauma CT scan and National Institute for Health and Care Excellence (NICE) guidelines suggest this should include a whole-body scanogram. This allows both the need for directed angiography and fracture imaging to be assessed and then images acquired at that first visit in a time-efficient manner. Whilst direct evidence is absent, indirect evidence favours reliance on hard signs (lack of pulses, expanding haematoma, continued bleeding) for making a prompt clinical diagnosis and avoiding time-consuming diagnostic tests that may alter the balance of ischaemic time on outcomes (4). All centres receiving these patients should have protocols in place for emergency referral for vascular assessment and reconstruction in collaboration with the orthopaedic team. Nevertheless, some injuries will not be salvageable. Where the patient is unconscious and a primary amputation must be performed in order to preserve life, the decision should be made by two consultants (2). One of the most difficult dilemmas is preparing an acutely injured conscious patient for the possibility of amputation. Patients must be made aware, as sensitively but unequivocally as possible, and consent obtained at primary exploration if necessary. If surgical exploration reveals the limb to be unsalvageable, the patient can be scheduled for delayed primary amputation following appropriate counselling and consent (4). The delayed primary amputation should be performed within 72 hours of injury and the decision to proceed down this route should be based on multidisciplinary assessment involving an orthopaedic surgeon, plastic surgeon, vascular specialist, rehabilitation specialist, the patient, and their family members or carers (4).

Ischaemia time

Physiological and preclinical studies reveal that muscle damage is present at 3 hours ischaemia time and is near complete, and irreversible, at 6 hours (6). The experimental data are corroborated by clinical series. In a series of 17 patients, all those with an ischaemic time of greater than 6 hours required amputation eventually whilst all limbs with an ischaemic time of less than 5 hours were salvaged (7). A meta-analysis of over 100 fractures with vascular injuries found that there was steep fall in limb salvage rate if the ischaemia time extended beyond 4 hours (8).

Vascular shunts

Popularised in 1971 (9), vascular shunts are used to establish flow to the devascularised limb prior to staged orthopaedic and vascular reconstruction (8–11). The surgical sequence of shunt rescue of the devascularised limb includes establishing proximal and distal control, intravascular lavage using heparinised saline (with Fogarty balloon catheterisation to re-establish flow if necessary), and the insertion of a shunt of a similar diameter to the traumatised vessel for a distance of 15–20 mm, which is then secured (12). Shunting has been shown to reduce complications, repeat operations, amputation rate, and duration of inpatient stay in a cohort of patients with blunt popliteal artery injuries and distal ischaemia (7). Shunting improves limb salvage where a major vascular injury is associated with high energy fractures (13,14). Shunting is well tolerated for vascular trauma in combat, avoiding the need for definitive revascularisation in austere environments (15). As well as revascularising the distal extremity, shunts minimise ongoing blood loss, combating the lethal triad of acidosis, coagulopathy, and hypothermia in the injured patient (11,12).

To avoid complicating the subsequent reconstruction of an associated open fracture, access incisions to enable shunting should be planned with the reconstruction in mind and preferably with the reconstructive surgeon present. Injuries to the popliteal vessels are best accessed via a curvilinear incision in the popliteal fossa that provides direct access above and below the site of vascular injury (16).

After shunting, the patient is stabilised and the limb is assessed with a view to salvage. Following skeletal stabilisation definitive vascular repair can be performed expeditiously using a reversed vein graft (17). Forearm veins are often superior to the saphenous vein as they can be harvested by a second team, tend to be the appropriate diameter, and are not as muscular as the saphenous and, hence, are less prone to spasm. The revascularised limb is at high risk of developing compartment syndrome and there should be a low threshold for decompression of all four compartments of the leg (Chapter 11).

Venous repair

Proximal venous injuries, including the femoral and popliteal, should be repaired at the same time as the arterial injuries. Whilst the collateral venous system may suffice in the short term, over time the poor venous return leads to the development of post-phlebitic changes (18). Proximal venous repairs are associated with high patency rates, with only venous repairs distal to the popliteal vein suffering from early thrombosis (18).

Nerve repair

A high index of suspicion for associated nerve injury is essential, especially in an unconscious patient. When a sharp nerve transection is encountered it should be ideally repaired at the same operation to avoid subsequent surgical exploration in the vicinity of the vascular repair and the accompanying scar tissue surrounding it (19). For larger nerves, knowledge of nerve topography and intraoperative fascicle stimulation are helpful to achieve anatomical approximation. If the nerve is sharply transected but with segmental loss, a interposition nerve graft is necessary (19). If, as is commonly the case, the nerve has suffered blunt trauma and/or when a primary repair is not possible, any directly observed or clinically inferred nerve injury must be documented along with any anatomic details that might facilitate safe delayed exploration and repair. A period of observation supplemented with nerve conduction studies and electromyography may be necessary to evaluate recovery when considering delayed exploration (19).

Ischaemia–reperfusion injury

Both muscle and nerve are highly sensitive to hypoxia, with histological evidence of tissue necrosis and reperfusion injury with 4 hours of warm ischaemia (6, 20–22). If the extremity was crushed, ischaemic effects may occur more quickly (23). Initially, muscle and nerve meet the ischaemic challenge by anaerobic respiration, incurring an oxygen debt. When saturated, this compromises membrane integrity and cellular homeostasis, which results in endothelial oedema leading to microcirculatory collapse and the 'no-reflow' phenomenon (6). Following restoration of microcirculatory flow, cell membrane peroxidation by superoxide free radicals results in the ischaemia–reperfusion injury, producing a systemic inflammatory response that may be life-threatening (24–26). Hence, surgeons must work closely with their anaesthetist colleagues to mitigate the adverse physiological consequences of delayed limb reperfusion.

Single-vessel leg

The prevalence of an occult vascular injury in lower extremity trauma is high, with one study noting that a third of injuries classified as Gustilo–Anderson grade IIIB had only one patent artery distal to the trifurcation (27). When planning soft tissue reconstruction, preoperative CT angiography may be useful, although this should be used with caution as it does not yield information about flow rate within the vessel or the status of the venae commitans. A review of patients with open fractures necessitating free flap coverage found that functional outcomes were significantly worse in the group with vascular injury compared with those with normal vasculature on angiography (28). A prospective randomised trial showed that repair of an occult vascular injury led to faster fracture union and lower infection rate (27). If the posterior tibial artery is injured, reconstruction should be considered. There is no contraindication to using a single patent artery as a recipient for end-to-side anastomosis for free tissue transfer with planning for a vascular reconstruction in place in case there are problems with the end-to-side anastomosis.

Outcomes

A systematic review and meta-analysis of the factors predictive of secondary amputation following lower extremity vascular trauma found that among a total of 3187 vascular repairs, an associated major soft tissue injury (OR 5.80), compartment syndrome (OR 5.11), multiple vessel trauma (OR 4.85), ischaemia exceeding 6 hours (OR 4.40), or an associated fracture (OR 4.30) were the factors most predictive of secondary amputation (29). A study of the United States National Trauma Databank revealed that of 1395 popliteal artery injuries, independent predictors of amputation included an associated fracture (OR 2.40), major soft tissue injury (OR 1.90), or nerve injury (OR 1.70) (30). In the largest individual study included in the meta-analysis (550 patients with 641 lower limb arterial injuries), failed attempted revascularisation (a factor not evaluated by the aforementioned studies) was found to be the single largest predictor of

secondary amputation (OR 16.70) (31). In a retrospective analysis of 58 patients with severe open tibial fractures requiring free tissue transfer, long-term
limb function, assessed using the Enneking score, was significantly worse in the
cohort of 18 with radiological evidence of a preoperative vascular injury (28).
Correspondingly, a randomised controlled trial of 157 Gustilo–Anderson IIIA
and IIIB fractures of the tibial shaft reported that repairing occult vascular injury reduced chronic swelling and atrophic skin changes, and improved power
and range of movement of the ankle (27).

Conclusion

The devascularised limb is a clinical emergency and optimal outcomes rely on
prompt identification and surgical exploration should adequate fracture reduction not result in restoration of circulation. CT angiography adds unnecessary
delay if performed as a stand-alone diagnostic test. Angiography can be use-
fully be obtained as part of a necessary whole body trauma CT. The site of injury
can be deduced usually from the three common fracture or dislocation patterns that produce vascular interruption. Prompt revascularisation is achieved
by the use of shunts. Limb viability and suitability for limb salvage can then be
assessed prior to skeletal stabilisation and definitive vascular reconstruction.
Injuries to major veins at the level of the popliteal fossa or proximally should
also be repaired. A low threshold for compartment decompression is advised.
In addition to failed revascularisation, concomitant major soft tissue injuries,
prolonged ischaemic time, and compartment syndrome are associated with
eventual amputation.

References

1. **Kragh, Jr. CJF, Walters TJ, Baer DG, Fox LCJ, Wade CE, Salinas J**, et al. Survival with emergency tourniquet use to stop bleeding in major limb trauma. Ann Surg. 2009;**249**:1–7.
2. **British Orthopaedic Association**. BOAST 6 : Management of arterial injuries associated with fractures and dislocations. London: BOA; 2014. https://www.boa.ac.uk/wp-content/uploads/2014/12/B
3. **Gustilo RB, Mendoza RM, Williams DN**. Problems in the management of type III (severe) open fractures: a new classification of type III open fractures. J Trauma. 1984;**24**:742–6.
4. **National Institute for Health and Care Excellence (NICE)**. Fractures (complex): assessment and management. London: National Institute for Health and Care Excellence (UK); 2016 https://www.nice.org.uk/guidance/ng37
5. **Ewing TE, Higgins GL, Perron AD, Strout TD**. Inter-rater reliability and false positive result rates of ankle brachial index measurements performed by emergency providers. Ann Emerg Med. 2010;**56**(3):S132–3.

6. **Blaisdell FW.** The pathophysiology of skeletal muscle ischemia and the reperfusion syndrome: a review. Cardiovasc Surg. 2002;**10**(6):620–30.

7. **Hossny A.** Blunt popliteal artery injury with complete lower limb ischemia: is routine use of temporary intraluminal arterial shunt justified? J Vasc Surg. 2004;**40**(1):61–6.

8. **Glass GE, Pearse MF, Nanchahal J.** Improving lower limb salvage following fractures with vascular injury: a systematic review and new management algorithm. J Plast Reconstr Aesthetic Surg. 2009;**62**(5):571–9.

9. **Eger M, Golcman L, Goldstein A, Hirsch M.** The use of a temporary shunt in the management of arterial vascular injuries. Surg Gynecol Obs. 1971;(131):67–70.

10. **Inaba K, Aksoy H, Seamon MJ, Marks JA, Duchesne J, Schroll R,** et al. Multicenter evaluation of temporary intravascular shunt use in vascular trauma. J Trauma Acute Care Surg. 2016;**80**(3):359–65.

11. **Subramanian A, Vercruysse G, Dente C, Wyrzykowski A, King E, Feliciano DV.** A decade's experience with temporary intravascular shunts at a civilian level I trauma center. J Trauma. 2008;**65**(2):316–24; discussion 324–6.

12. **Hornez E, Boddaert G, Ngabou UD, Aguir S, Baudoin Y, Mocellin N,** et al. Temporary vascular shunt for damage control of extremity vascular injury: a toolbox for trauma surgeons. J Visc Surg. 2015;**152**(6):363–8.

13. **McHenry TP, Holcomb JB, Aoki N, Lindsey RW.** Fractures with major vascular injuries from gunshot wounds: implications of surgical sequence. J Trauma. 2002;**53**(4):717–21.

14. **Desai PP, Audige L, Suk M.** Combined orthopedic and vascular lower extremity injuries: sequence of care and outcomes. Am J Orthop. 2012;**41**(4):182–6.

15. **Rasmussen TE, Clouse WD, Jenkins DH, Peck M a, Eliason JL, Smith DL.** The use of temporary vascular shunts as a damage control adjunct in the management of wartime vascular injury. J Trauma. 2006;**61**(1):8–12; discussion 12–15.

16. **Feliciano D V.** Pitfalls in the management of peripheral vascular injuries. Trauma Surg Acute Care Open. 2017;**2**(1):e000110. http://tsaco.bmj.com/lookup/doi/10.1136/tsaco-2017-000110

17. **Veith FJ, Gupta SK, Ascer E, White-flores S, Samson RH, Scher LA,** et al. Six-year prospective multicenter randomized comparison of autologous saphenous vein and expanded polytetrafluoroethylene grafts in infrainguinal arterial reconstructions. J Vasc Surg. 1986;**3**:104–14.

18. **Kuralay E, Demirkiliç U, Özal E, Öz BS, Cingöz F, Gunay C,** et al. A quantitative approach to lower extremity vein repair. J Vasc Surg. 2002;**36**(6):1213–18.

19. **Ray WZ, MacKinnon SE.** Management of nerve gaps: autografts, allografts, nerve transfers, and end-to-side neurorrhaphy. Exp Neurol. 2010;**223**(1):77–85.

20. **Labbe R, Lindsay T, Walker PM.** The extent and distribution of skeletal muscle necrosis after graded periods of complete ischemia. J Vasc Surg. 1987;**6**(2):152–7.

21. **Kinoshita Y, Monafo WW.** Nerve and muscle blood flow during hindlimb ischemia and reperfusion in rats. J Neurosurg. 1994;**80**(6):1078–84.

22. **Rorabeck CH.** Tourniquet-induced nerve ischaemia: an experimental investigation. J Trauma. 1980;**20**(4):280–6.

23. **Criswell TL, Corona BT, Ward CL, Miller M, Patel M, Wang Z,** et al. Compression-induced muscle injury in rats that mimics compartment syndrome in humans. Am J Pathol. 2012;**180**(2):787–97.

24. **Kerrigan CL, Stotland MA.** Ischemia reperfusion injury: a review. Microsurgery. 1993;**14**(3):165–75.

25. **Siemionow M, Arslan E.** Ischemia/reperfusion injury: a review in relation to free tissue transfers. Microsurgery. 2004;**24**(6):468–75.

26. **Gillani S, Cao J, Suzuki T, Hak DJ.** The effect of ischemia reperfusion injury on skeletal muscle. Injury. 2012;**43**(6):670–5.

27. **Waikakul S, Sakkarnkosol S, Vanadurongwan V.** Vascular injuries in compound fractures of the leg with initially adequate circulation. J Bone Joint Surg. 1998;**80**(2):254–8.

28. **Chummun S, Wigglesworth TA, Young K, Healey B, Wright TC, Chapman TWL,** et al. Does vascular injury affect the outcome of open tibial fractures? Plast Reconstr Surg. 2013;**131**(2):303–9.

29. **Perkins ZB, Yet B, Glasgow S, Cole E, Marsh W, Brohi K,** et al. Meta-analysis of prognostic factors for amputation following surgical repair of lower extremity vascular trauma. Br J Surg. 2015;**102**(5):436–50.

30. **Mullenix PS, Steele SR, Andersen CA, Starnes BW, Salim A, Martin MJ.** Limb salvage and outcomes among patients with traumatic popliteal vascular injury: an analysis of the National Trauma Data Bank. J Vasc Surg. 2006;**44**(1):94–100.

31. **Hafez HM, Woolgar J, Robbs J V.** Lower extremity arterial injury: results of 550 cases and review of risk factors associated with limb loss. J Vasc Surg. 2001;**33**(6):1212–19.

Chapter 11

Compartment Syndrome in the Lower Limb

Summary

1. Compartment syndrome is a surgical emergency and must be diagnosed and treated promptly.
2. Accurate diagnosis of the condition relies of the collation of clinical features and intracompartmental pressure measurements. Serial assessments can help establish the diagnosis when there is uncertainty.
3. Unrelenting pain out of proportion to the injury, paraesthesia or paresis of nerves within the affected compartments, and passive stretch exacerbation of pain are important clinical features.
4. Threshold for diagnosis in adults when using compartment pressure measurements is a perfusion pressure (diastolic blood pressure—intracompartmental pressure) of less than 30 mmHg for 2 consecutive hours.
5. Decompression in the leg is performed using the two-incision technique. The posteromedial incision is 12–15 mm posterior to the posteromedial border and the anterior incision 2 cm lateral to the crest of the tibia. All four compartments are to be released adequately to enable extrusion of enlarged muscle.
6. All non-viable muscle is excised and fasciotomy wounds covered immediately with meshed split skin grafts or within 72 hours at the latest.

Introduction

Acute compartment syndrome of the limb is characterised by ischaemia of the soft tissues in association with raised tissue pressures within unyielding osseofascial compartments. It is a surgical emergency as the sustained high levels of pressure compromise capillary perfusion lead to hypoxia-induced death of tissue. Compartment syndrome may occur following a fracture or revascularisation of an ischaemic limb; sometimes it is associated with a crush injury (1). Irreversible muscle and nerve damage occur when hypoxic levels are sustained and the period beyond which the damage becomes permanent depends on the type of tissue and pressure levels. Consequently, prompt diagnosis and decompression may save limbs. A missed diagnosis is associated with significant morbidity arising from the ischaemic necrosis and, sometimes, putrefaction of tissues within the compartment. Late decompression, after the stage when tissue can be rescued, should be avoided because of the risks of infection and reperfusion injury.

The principles described in the foregoing account apply to the upper and lower limb except for the hand and foot.

Making the diagnosis

An increased awareness of the condition, particularly with some fracture types, and repeated clinical assessments and intracompartmental pressure measurements will enable early diagnosis and treatment. Heightened vigilance is recommended for young adults with mid-diaphyseal tibial fractures, tibial plateau fractures, or proximal tibial fractures associated with knee dislocation (2, 3). These injury types have a higher association with acute compartment syndrome, possibly from the high-energy nature of the underlying mechanisms producing greater soft tissue disruption. The key to making an accurate diagnosis is the serial collation of signs and symptoms. The greater the number of positive features, the more likely is the diagnosis to be accurate, especially if this is repeated over a short period of observation. Whilst a single positive finding has a probability of an accurate diagnosis of 25%, three findings increase this probability to 93% (4).

An important feature of compartment syndrome in the conscious patient is severe pain that is out of proportion to the injury and that fails to improve in the expected time course after surgery or after a judicious dose of analgesics. The pain is exacerbated by passive stretching of the muscles of the affected compartment but this sign is not valuable in children, who are influenced by apprehension and fear of pain. The classic five Ps of compartment syndrome (pain, pallor, paraesthesia, pulselessness, and paralysis) are not relevant to an early diagnosis of the condition; if anything, waiting for all five Ps would inevitably lead to a late diagnosis. Of the five, pain, paraesthesia, and weakness (paralysis) are likely to be found early and a clinical examination should look for signs of nerve impairment, e.g. sensory loss within the areas supplied by nerves traversing the involved compartments. In the lower leg the anterior compartment is most commonly involved and numbness in the first web space (deep peroneal nerve) is an early sign.

The clinical signs of compartment syndrome are affected if nerve blocks or regional anaesthesia has been used or if the patient is unconscious. The impediment introduced by such effective analgesic methods is not about the ability to make the diagnosis but about making the diagnosis early. Eliciting clinical signs can be difficult in non-compliant patients and young children. In such scenarios, continuous measurement of intracompartmental pressure has its advocates (5). In the unconscious or non-compliant patient, it may be the only available clinical parameter. The pressure is measured using purpose-made devices, which are solid state transducer intracompartmental catheters (STIC, Stryker, USA) or transducer-tipped catheters (Omnibar E5F, Raumedic, Germany). Both produce similar readings but single measurements should be used cautiously; corroborative clinical signs or repeated measurements help add weight to the diagnosis of compartment syndrome (6). The commonly used threshold for decompression in adults is when the perfusion pressure (diastolic pressure minus intracompartmental pressure) is less than 30 mmHg, especially when sustained for more than 2 hours. In a consecutive series of over 900 adults with tibial fractures, the sensitivity and specificity for making the diagnosis with this threshold were 94% and 98%, respectively, and led to fasciotomies in 18% (5). The balance between a prompt diagnosis and unnecessary fasciotomy can be difficult; both untreated compartment syndrome and unneeded surgery carry morbidity (7–9). Additionally, this perfusion pressure threshold can be unsuitable for young children who have diastolic blood pressures between 40 and 55 mmHg (this would suggest intracompartmental pressures of 10–25 mmHg would then prompt a fasciotomy). The incidence of acute compartment syndrome is lower in young children (<12 years) and may occur as late as 65 hours after injury (10). The recommendation for young children is to use serial clinical examination repeated over brief intervals whilst the limb is nursed flat and to note if there has been a record of increasing analgesic needs (11, 12).

Treatment

Surgery to decompress the four compartments in the leg is the only treatment available; whilst preparing for surgery it is prudent to confirm that all circumferential dressings have been divided. Long incisions through skin and fascia are needed to decompress adequately and allow extrusion of the increased muscle bulk. Subcutaneous incisions in the fascia through shorter skin incisions are not recommended (13). We recommend the two-incision technique (14, 15). The positions of the incisions are different from classic descriptions (16); this represents a deliberate attempt to facilitate soft tissue cover of open fractures by preserving perforators arising from axial vessels such that local fasciocutaneous flap options remain viable (Figure 11.1a–d). There are added advantages: the

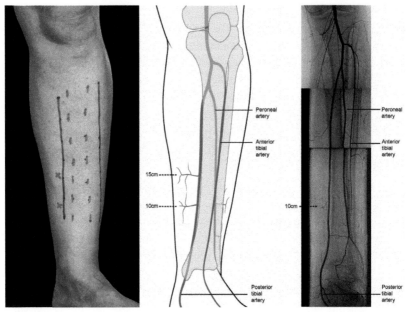

Figure 11.1 Placement of the recommended two-incision fasciotomy in compartment syndrome or wound extensions for wound excision in open fractures of the tibia. (a) The posteromedial border and tibial crest are marked in green. The fasciotomy incisions are in blue, located 12–15 mm posterior to the posteromedial border and 2 cm lateral to the crest. The red crosses mark out the location of perforators arising from the posterior tibial artery; the posteromedial incision must lie anterior to these perforating vessels. (b) Line drawing showing the perforators from the posterior and anterior tibial arteries. Their approximate levels proximal to the medial and lateral malleoli, respectively, are marked. (c) Montage of an arteriogram. The 10 cm perforator on the medial side is usually the largest and most reliable for distally based fasciocutaneous flaps. In this patient the anterior tibial artery had been disrupted after an open dislocation of the ankle—this accounts for the poor flow seen in that vessel. The distances the perforators are located proximal to the tip of the medial malleolus are approximate and can vary. Preserving the perforators can be achieved with this two-incision technique and it is important to avoid placing incisions that cross between perforators.

incisions provide good access to the posterior and anterior tibial vessels should these be needed as recipient vessels for free flaps.

The superficial and deep posterior compartments are decompressed by an incision placed 12–15 mm just posterior to the posteromedial border of the tibia. At times the posteromedial border is difficult to palpate in the swollen limb but starting from the medial malleolus (a bony landmark always felt even in such scenarios) it is possible to gauge the position with some accuracy. The placement

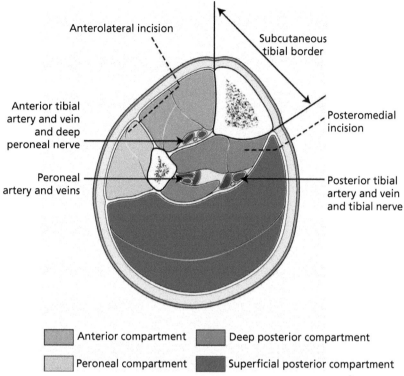

Figure 11.2 Cross-section through the middle of the leg showing the incisions for decompressing all four compartments. The medial incision is 12–15 mm posterior to the posteromedial border of the tibia and the lateral 2 cm lateral to the crest. The lateral incision continues subfascially to reach the peroneal septum, which is then divided.

of this posteromedial fasciotomy incision is 12 mm from the posteromedial border of the tibia in children but closer to 15 mm when the patient is an adult. As a guide, if the child's leg is approximately the size of an adult forearm, the distance of 12 mm should be used; as the limb approaches adult size, then the 15 mm distance is safe. The posterior tibial neurovascular bundle lies between the muscles of the two posterior compartments, just next to the investing fascia of the deep compartment. Care must be taken when decompressing this compartment from the posteromedial side. Proximally, the soleus originates from the posteromedial border of the tibia and needs to be taken down sharply to allow full access to the fascia of the deep posterior compartment.

The anterior and lateral (peroneal) compartments are decompressed by an incision 2 cm lateral to the crest of the tibia. Entry into the anterior compartment is immediate but the peroneal compartment is decompressed by retracting the muscles of the anterior compartment medially and identifying the septum separating anterior and lateral muscle groups and incising it carefully. This septum can be seen and felt lateral to the fibula. The surface anatomy—tibial crest and posteromedial border—for the placement of the two skin incisions can be difficult to define in a swollen limb but careful palpation will reveal these contours.

There has been a resurgence of interest in single incision fasciotomies for decompression of all four compartments (17, 18). We do not advocate the technique: reaching all four compartments from a single lateral incision involves undermining the skin anteriorly and posteriorly. This degloves the skin and can pose potential problems for wound healing in a zone of injury. The two-incision technique decompresses by allowing the greater volume of contents (muscle) within the compartments to spill out and thereby occupy a larger space.

Muscle viability must be checked after compartment decompression and excised if necrotic. If all devitalised tissue is removed, we favour immediate coverage with meshed, split thickness grafts secured with a negative pressure foam dressing using pressures of 50–70 mmHg only. This provides cover to the wounds and fracture with immediate effect. If closure is to be delayed because of uncertainty over tissue viability, a temporary dressing is applied (19). Return to theatre for final inspection, wound excision, and definitive fracture cover should be accomplished within 72 hours.

A late diagnosis of compartment syndrome and subsequent fasciotomy can lead to severe infection, renal failure and death (20–22). The definition of late diagnosis is unclear and there is evidence that even by 3 hours after trauma there is muscle necrosis (23). This suggests there may be varying degrees of the condition and that our current tools for establishing the diagnosis—whether clinical features or pressure measurements—are surrogates for the cell death occurring from impaired tissue perfusion. Newer modalities are being investigated and include near-infrared spectrometry and tissue ultrafiltration samples (24); at present, clinical examination and compartment pressure measurement remain at the forefront of diagnosis (25).

There is controversy over how best to manage a late presentation of compartment syndrome in adults as decompression enables reperfusion of necrotic muscle and leads to a rhabdomyolysis syndrome. Leaving the compartments closed will allow the necrosis to complete without reperfusion; this may be a safer prospect (26). Conversely there are those who advocate decompression even if the diagnosis is late but with removal of necrotic muscle (to the extent of compartment removal, if necessary, leaving the traversing neurovascular bundles intact). There is insufficient evidence to provide clear guidance but a late decompression without removal of necrotic muscle will lead to greater morbidity, and potentially death, from reperfusion and rhabdomyolysis.

This contrasts with the situation when dealing with children where the syndrome may evolve more slowly and result in a late diagnosis; serial assessments are advised and fasciotomy, even when late, can be associated with recovery (27).

Conclusion

Acute compartment syndrome can occur in open tibial fractures; there is no spontaneous decompression of the compartments from the wound. The diagnosis involves vigilance, repeated clinical assessments and intracompartmental pressure measurements. Treatment is by a dual-incision fasciotomy and decompression of all four compartments of the tibia. Wound excision must follow if non-viable tissue is identified.

References

1. **McQueen M, Gaston P., Court-Brown C.** Acute compartment syndrome: who is at risk? J Bone Joint Surg Br. 2000;**82-B**(2):200–3.
2. **Weinlein J, Schmidt A.** Acute compartment syndrome in tibial plateau fractures—beware! J Knee Surg.2010;**23**(1):9–16.
3. **Park S, Ahn J, Gee, AO, Kuntz AF, Esterhai, JL.** Compartment syndrome in tibial fractures. J Orthop Trauma. 2009;**23**(7):514–18.
4. **Ulmer T.** The clinical diagnosis of compartment syndrome of the lower leg: are clinical findings predictive of the disorder? J Orthop Trauma. 2002;**16**(8):572–7.
5. **McQueen MM, Duckworth AD, Aitken SA, Court-Brown CM.** The estimated sensitivity and specificity of compartment pressure monitoring for acute compartment syndrome. J Bone Joint Surg Am. 2013;**95**(8):673–7.
6. **Collinge C., Kuper M.** Comparison of three methods for measuring intracompartmental pressure in injured limbs of trauma patients. J Orthop Trauma. 2010;**24**(6):364–8.
7. **Janzing HMJ, Broos PLO.** Routine monitoring of compartment pressure in patients with tibial fractures: beware of overtreatment! Injury. 2001;**32**(5):415–21.
8. **Giannoudis PV, Nicolopoulos C, Dinopoulos H, Ng A, Adedapo S.** The impact of lower leg compartment syndrome on health related quality of life. Injury. 2002;**33**(2):117–21.
9. **Fitzgerald AM, Gaston P, Wilson Y, Quaba A, McQueen MM** Long-term sequelae of fasciotomy wounds. Br J Plast Surg. 2000;**53**(8):690–3.
10. **Ferlic PW, Singer G, Kraus T, Eberl R.** The acute compartment syndrome following fractures of the lower leg in children. Injury. 2012;**43**(10):1743–6.
11. **Al-Dadah OQ, Darrah C, Cooper A, Donell ST, Patel AD.** Continuous compartment pressure monitoring vs. clinical monitoring in tibial diaphyseal fractures. Injury. 2008;**39**(10):1204–9.
12. **Noonan, KJ, McCarthy JJ.** Compartment syndromes in the pediatric patient. J Ped Orthop. 2010;**30**:S96–101.

13. **Cohen MS, Garfin SR, Hargens AR, Mubarak SJ.** Acute compartment syndrome. Effect of dermotomy on fascial decompression in the leg. J Bone Joint Surg Br. 1991;**73-B**(2):287–90.

14. **Pearse MF, Harry L, Nanchahal J.** Acute compartment syndrome of the leg: fasciotomies must be performed early, but good surgical technique is important. (Editorial). BMJ. 2002;**325**(7364):557.

15. **Nanchahal J, Nayagam S, Khan U, Moran C, Barrett S, Sanderson F, Pallister I.** Standards for the Management of Open Fractures of the Lower Limb, ed. H Laing. London: Royal Society of Medicine Press Ltd; 2009, p. 112.

16. **Mubarak SJ, Owen CA.** Double-incision fasciotomy of the leg for decompression in compartment syndromes. J Bone Joint Surg Am. 1977;**59**(2):184–7.

17. **Masquelet AC.** Acute compartment syndrome of the leg: pressure measurement and fasciotomy. Orthop Traumatol: SurgRes. 2010;**96**(8):913–17.

18. **Bible JE, McClure DJ, Mir HR.** Analysis of single-incision versus dual-incision fasciotomy for tibial fractures with acute compartment syndrome. J Orthop Trauma. 2013;**27**(11):607–11.

19. **Acosta S, Bjorck M, Wanhainen A.** Negative-pressure wound therapy for prevention and treatment of surgical-site infections after vascular surgery. Br J Surg. 2017;**104**(2):e75–84.

20. **Finkelstein JA, Hunter GA, Hu RW.** Lower limb compartment syndrome: course after delayed fasciotomy. J Trauma. 1996;**40**(3):342–4.

21. **Shaw CJ, Spencer JD.** Late management of compartment syndromes. Injury. 1995;**26**(9):633–5.

22. **Chatzizisis YS, Misirli G, Hatzitolios AI, Giannoglou GD.** The syndrome of rhabdomyolysis: complications and treatment. Eur J Intern Med. 2008;**19**(8):568–74.

23. **Vaillancourt C, Shrier I, Vandal A, Falk M, Rossignol M, Vernec A, Somogyi D.** Acute compartment syndrome: how long before muscle necrosis occurs? Cjem. 2004;**6**(3):147–54.

24. **Harvey EJ, Sanders DW, Shuler MS, Lawendy AR, Cole AL, Alqahtani SM, Schmidt AH.** What's new in acute compartment syndrome? J Orthop Trauma. 2012;**26**(12):699–702.

25. **Schmidt AH.** Acute compartment syndrome. Orthop Clin North Am. 2016;**47**(3):517–25.

26. **Glass GE, Staruch RM, Simmons J, Lawton G, Nanchahal J, Jain A, Hettiaratchy SP.** Managing missed lower extremity compartment syndrome in the physiologically stable patient: a systematic review and lessons from a Level I trauma center. J Trauma Acute Care Surg. 2016;**81**(2):380–7.

27. **Flynn JM, Bashyal RK, Yeger-McKeever M, Garner MR, Launay F, Sponseller PD.** Acute traumatic compartment syndrome of the leg in children: diagnosis and outcome. J Bone Joint Surg Am. 2011;**93**(10):937–41.

Chapter 12

Amputation

Summary

1. Primary amputation is associated with similar long-term outcomes to limb salvage and should be considered a reconstructive procedure.

2. The decision to amputate or salvage a limb is based on a careful multidisciplinary analysis of both injury and patient variables and should not be based on an injury severity score tool. The decision to amputate after trauma must involve an orthopaedic surgeon, a plastic surgeon, a rehabilitation specialist, and the patient and their family members or carers whenever possible. Operative photographs illustrating the extent of limb injury should be obtained and stored in the patient's file.

3. Immediate amputation is indicated in the following cases:

   a) when a limb is the source of uncontrollable life-threatening bleeding or as part of damage control in cases of severe limb trauma in unstable polytraumatised patients;

   b) an avascular limb with a warm ischaemia time greater than 4–6 hours;

   c) extensive crush injuries, particularly involving both the tibia and the ipsilateral foot.

4. Positive neurological findings at presentation including absent plantar sensation and lack of motor function are not absolute indicators for amputation but may warrant direct nerve visualisation.

5. When indicated, a delayed primary amputation should be performed within 72 hours of the injury.

6. Maximising residual limb length is imperative for mobility. A through-the-knee level should be considered in preference to above-knee, and soft tissue reconstructive techniques should be used where there is sufficient bone but inadequate soft tissues to achieve a more distal amputation level.

7. Vigilant follow-up with emphasis on the whole patient including pain management, psychological health, and active rehabilitation is essential to maximise good functional outcomes. Revision surgery can dramatically improve prosthetic use, limb function, and quality of life, and regular orthoplastic review should continue for at least 2 years.

Introduction

The decision to amputate rather than reconstruct a severely injured limb ('mangled extremity') has historically been one of the most difficult choices faced by a trauma surgeon. The surgeon's responsibility is heightened by the knowledge that delayed or incorrect decision-making may lead to worse outcomes (1). Unfortunately, hard data upon which to base reliable decisions remain elusive. A prospective analysis of the use of scoring systems including the Limb Salvage Index, the Predictive Salvage Index, the Hanover Fracture Scale, and the NISSSA (Nerve injury, Ischaemia, Soft-tissue contamination, Skeletal damage, Shock, Age) and MESS (Mangled Extremity Severity Score) scores did not validate the clinical utility of any of the scoring algorithms (2, 3).

A number of studies, including two meta-analyses, have shown the final outcomes of amputation after trauma are similar to the outcomes after limb salvage, with high rates of long-term disability reported in both patient groups (4–6). More recent research has focused on injury and patient factors that may impact on the final functional outcome after both amputation and limb salvage (1, 6, 7). We advocate early identification of poor prognostic factors as the basis for the decision to amputate or salvage.

Resuscitation and limb assessment

A severe limb-threatening injury is usually obvious and can be a distraction to the assessment and resuscitation of the patient. Up to 17% of patients with severe limb trauma will have associated life-threatening injuries, which must be identified and treated according to the advanced trauma life support (ATLS) principles of ABCDE (Airway, Breathing, Circulation, Disability, Exposure) (8), but also consider that the limb injury itself may be life-threatening. A thorough limb examination is only performed after the airway is secured and the cardiopulmonary function is stable. Haemorrhage from the limb is traditionally assessed during C (Circulation) of the primary survey and is addressed by either direct pressure or the judicious use of a tourniquet. However, more recently, the need to deal with catastrophic haemorrhage at an earlier stage has been recognised in the sequence CABCDE.

Immediate primary amputation

There are a number of uncommon injury scenarios when immediate amputation is indicated. Incomplete traumatic amputation involving almost complete severance of the limb, often accompanied by extensive injury to the distal segment, requires prompt surgical completion of the amputation. Extensive crush injuries involving both the tibia and the foot and avascular limbs with a warm ischaemic time in excess of 4–6 hours also demand early amputation. Occasionally, unstable polytraumatised patients may need urgent amputation of uncontrolled bleeding mangled extremities as part of a damage control protocol when the patient's general condition precludes the lengthy reconstruction required for salvage (3). Operative photographs are valuable documentary evidence of the extent of the limb injury and should be taken and stored in the patient's record (9).

Guillotine amputations are to be avoided as they sacrifice residual limb length and viable tissue. Viable muscle and skin flaps should be retained whenever possible (10). Wounds should not be formally closed and the use of negative-pressure wound therapy dressings is recommended. If immediate amputation is required for life-threatening injuries, complete documentation of the extent of the injury with intra-operative photographs will be helpful in explaining the decision to the patient and their family.

Decision-making variables

The decision to amputate or reconstruct a severely injured extremity should be based on an analysis of the characteristics of the limb injury and the physiological reserve of the patient (Box 12.1). A multidisciplinary discussion involving an orthopaedic surgeon, a plastic surgeon, rehabilitation specialist, the patient, and their family or carers is essential whenever possible before embarking on surgery. A recent meta-analysis of prognostic factors associated with amputation following repair of lower extremity vascular trauma highlighted a number of factors associated with an increased risk of secondary amputation (11). Risk factors for amputation included major soft tissue injury, compartment syndrome, an ischaemic time beyond 6 hours and age over 55 years.

Limb ischaemia

Reperfusion of an ischaemic limb needs to be achieved within 4–6 hours of injury (see Chapter 10). However, the precise time of injury may not have been established and the ischaemic threshold may be reduced if the patient has been persistently hypotensive (12).

Neurological injury

Historically, the absence of plantar sensation in the traumatised limb was considered an indication for amputation due to risk of development of neuropathic ulcers and other chronic complications associated with an insensate foot. However, a study comparing patients presenting with an insensate foot

Box 12.1 Decision-making variables

Amputation or limb salvage

Decision-making variables

Injury variables

- vascular trauma and warm ischaemia time
- uncontrolled bleeding
- neurological trauma
- ipsilateral foot trauma
- soft tissue trauma
- contamination
- bone loss

Patient variables

- multiple injuries (Injury Severity Score, ISS)
- haemodynamic shock
- age
- smoking
- medical co-morbidities
- occupation
- social and cultural

on clinical examination had similar outcomes following limb salvage at over 2 and a half years compared to a matched group with intact plantar sensibility at presentation (13). The presence of abnormal neurological findings at presentation, either motor or sensory, remains a significant finding and the nerve should be inspected at the initial wound excision, particularly in the presence of suspected arterial trauma. Confirmed irreversible nerve trauma, particularly of the posterior tibial nerve due to avulsion, transection, or segmental loss in an adult should be factored into the decision whether to salvage or amputate the limb.

Soft tissue damage and contamination

The level and the extent of soft tissue damage directly influences the surgical options for both amputation and limb salvage, and is a major factor in determining the functional potential of the limb. Soft tissue damage may be caused by the injury, ischaemia, or by compartment syndrome. Localised muscle damage can be offset by muscle transfers, e.g. transfer of tibialis posterior for peroneal or anterior compartment muscle loss. However, more extensive muscle loss, particularly affecting the posterior compartment muscles, usually results in poor final function and amputation should be considered. Severe wound contamination is often associated with major soft tissue loss because of the need for aggressive and repeated wound excision.

Extensive soft tissue damage almost inevitably results in a scarred and atrophic limb with compromised function and an early amputation may be in the best long-term interest of the patient.

Associated foot and ankle trauma.

Severe open tibial fractures are occasionally associated with ipsilateral crush injuries of the foot and ankle. A high proportion of patients continue to have neuropathic pain and poor function despite successful salvage and treatment of crush-type foot injuries (14). Studies of multiply injured patients with foot injuries found significantly worse functional outcome scores compared with those without foot injuries (15, 16). Based on these data, amputation may provide better long-term functional outcomes in patients presenting with a severe open tibial fracture and concomitant severe ipsilateral foot trauma.

Bone loss

Extensive bone defects can be successfully managed by a number of techniques, including autogenous bone grafting, vascularised fibula grafts, or distraction osteogenesis (see Chapter 9). However, the healing index (number of months of treatment per centimetre of new bone) is high. A 5 cm defect can be successfully restored by distraction osteogenesis over approximately 8–9 months. Reconstruction of larger bone defects will take over 12 months and involve multiple operations. In addition, the patient will need to be compliant, motivated, have good social support, and ideally a non-smoker. By contrast, a successful unilateral trans-tibial amputee will be walking largely unaided at around 3–4 months and will be fully ambulant at around 5–6 months.

Smoking

In addition to being a marker for medical co-morbidities such as coronary heart disease and obstructive airway disease, cigarette smoking is also a prognostic variable influencing both bone and soft tissue healing. Data from the Lower Extremity Assessment Project (LEAP) study demonstrated that current smokers with limb-threatening open tibial fractures were 37% less likely to achieve union than non-smokers, and 3.7 times more likely to develop osteomyelitis than non-smokers (17). Similar results were reported in a recent systemic review, which found smoking significantly increased the overall risk for non-union, particularly in tibial and open fractures (18). Smoking may also adversely affect soft tissue reconstruction. Two recent meta-analyses have revealed significantly increased risks of cutaneous necrosis, delayed wound healing, and surgical site infections in smokers (19, 20).

Timing of delayed primary amputation

In practice, most severe limb injuries are suitable for staged management. Marginally viable tissue may take hours to demarcate and an evolving injury can be definitively declared unsalvageable at 48 hours. A staged approach also allows time to investigate the patient's general welfare and counsel the patient and their family on the implications of their injury. Involvement of a multidisciplinary limb rehabilitation team is crucial, including patients who have completed their rehabilitation.

Once the decision has been reached, amputation should be performed as soon as possible and within 72 hours of injury (3).

Common injury scenarios where delayed primary amputation should be considered include a major open tibia fracture with a severe foot injury, segmental bone loss involving more than a third of the tibial shaft, loss of two or more muscle compartments, and an ischaemia limb with a proven nerve injury.

Residual limb reconstruction

The aim of residual limb ('stump') reconstruction is the preservation of maximal limb length whilst ensuring adequate soft tissue cover (1). Maintaining length in the presence of widespread tissue damage is a major challenge and in practice the most distal level of viable soft tissue dictates the amputation length. Amputation at the level of the fracture site should be avoided if viable distal bone is present, and proximal fractures should be managed with standard fixation techniques (21). The bone ends should be beveled to remove jagged edges, which may cause local discomfort. The construction of a bone bridge between the tibia and shortened fibular (Ertl technique) has been proposed for younger amputees but conflicting data are present in the literature and comparative studies are lacking (1, 22).

Soft tissue reconstruction aims to provide durable and comfortable padding over the bone ends, and to restore muscular control of the leg (1). A sound myodesis is essential to maintain mechanical limb alignment and optimise muscular control of the residual leg. Detached muscle groups should be secured under physiological tension to the distal bone through drill holes using stout sutures. Standard myocutaneous flaps, such as a long posterior flap for trans-tibial amputation are not usually available and 'flaps of opportunity' are used to reconstruct the soft tissue envelope. Skin grafting and tissue transfer with pedicled or free flaps may be required to maximise residual limb length. However, skin grafts and scar tissue do not withstand the shear forces associated with prosthetic wear and length preservation should not be at the expense of inadequate soft tissue cover, which may preclude successful limb fitting. Suture lines and compromised integument should also be avoided at key weight-bearing locations on the residual limb.

Neuroma formation is inevitable following nerve transection but is usually asymptomatic unless exposed to mechanical stimulation. Named nerves should be identified, gently handled, cut sharply, and allowed to retract proximally to lie well away from the weight-bearing area. The sural nerve should be identified during trans-tibial surgery because of the high risk for inclusion in the suture line. However, every effort should be made to avoid injury to cutaneous nerves to maintain the sensibility of cutaneous flaps.

The use of a tourniquet is recommended to reduce blood loss and transfusion requirements (23) but the tourniquet should be deflated before closure to allow an assessment of tissue perfusion and aid effective haemostasis. The use of drains may be considered to limit postoperative hematoma formation.

Improving amputation outcomes

Amputation is a life-changing event and the most important issue for amputees is their quality of life after treatment. Disability and poor outcomes can be significantly improved by a number of therapeutic interventions delivered in a multidisciplinary setting (1, 6, 22, 24).

Amputation level

Trans-tibial (below-knee) amputations are associated with superior outcomes compared with more proximal amputations and every effort must be made to preserve the knee, including vascular repair or flap coverage. Occasionally, short trans-tibial residual limbs can be avoided if the foot remnant is not traumatised by raising a pedicled flap of plantar skin and calcaneus and securing it to the end of the divided tibia (25).

If a trans-tibial level is not possible, through-the-knee amputation (TKA) should be considered, particularly if there is a viable posterior myofasciocutaneous flap to provide good soft tissue coverage for the residual limb. The advantages of a TKA over an above-knee amputation (AKA) in ambulatory patients include an end weight-bearing residual limb, enhanced proprioception, preserved adductor muscle insertion, a longer lever arm, and decreased metabolic cost of ambulation compared with AKA (26, 27). The Gritti–Stokes modification of knee disarticulation may offer improved weight-bearing characteristics in the trauma patient (27). In patients unlikely to ambulate, a TKA maximises ease of transfers because the limb is end-bearing and facilitates wheelchair mobility by providing better counterbalance due to the longer residual limb (26).

Although the LEAP study reported poor outcomes in a small cohort of 18 patients, a recent meta-analysis of 27 studies comprising 3105 traumatic amputees including 104 TKA, revealed significantly superior Physical Component Scores in patients with TKA compared with trans-femoral amputees (6). In addition, the proportion of TKA patients who could walk at least 500 m was slightly greater than patients with trans-tibial amputations and significantly more than trans-femoral amputees.

However, the study also found that patients with a TKA wore their prostheses significantly less and reported significantly more pain than those with trans-femoral amputation, which was attributed to potential suboptimal soft tissue coverage and prosthetic fitting difficulties (6). TKA is also associated with knee-level asymmetry, most marked when seated and the lower knee joint axis may complicate gait training. It has been suggested that the greater length of the TKA provides a superior lever arm, which confers greater mobility than a trans-femoral amputation, with less impact on the quality of life (6). TKA currently represents <5% of traumatic civilian amputees and the relative lack of experience with the surgical technique and in caring for patients with a TKA may explain some of the pain and limb-fitting issues and outcomes may be further improved by developments in TKA prosthetic design (6).

Infection

Infection is the commonest complication after severe extremity trauma and developed in 34% of the patients undergoing primary amputation in the LEAP study (28). Predisposing factors for infection in the LEAP included diabetes, injury severity, and smoking (17). A higher rate of infection was also reported following delay in performing the primary amputation (29). The highest rate of wound infection in the LEAP study was seen after late amputation with 17 out of 25 patients (68%) experiencing a wound infection and 10 patients developed osteomyelitis (40%). The National Institute for Health and Care Excellence (NICE) recommend that delayed primary amputation should be performed within 72 hours of the injury.

The diagnosis of residual limb infection is predominantly clinical and is characterised by local inflammation and increased drainage. Management is primarily surgical, with prompt drainage of fluid collections and aggressive wound excision of necrotic and devascularised tissue with multiple operative biopsies for microbial analysis. Empiric broad-spectrum antibiotics covering nosocomial organisms should be administered pending culture results (29, 30).

Pain

Pain is a common cause of disability after traumatic amputation (1, 31). Phantom limb pain affects 50–80% of amputees and, although the pathogeneses is not completely understood, the development of cortical pain memories is considered important (32). Pre-amputation and residual limb pain plus psychological factors such as emotional stress and anxiety probably all contribute to the development of phantom limb pain (6). Early administration of effective analgesia as soon after injury as possible will not only control acute pain but may also reduce the risk of chronic pain. Pre-emptive analgesia is also indicated to prevent the establishment of central sensitisation and pain memories evoked by surgery and early mobilisation. Although a randomised study of epidural anaesthesia for elective amputation cases showed no benefit (32), the analgesia was not truly pre-emptive as central nervous system changes may have already been established and epidural anaesthesia may have a role in acute pain management.

Psychological response

An intense emotional response following traumatic amputation is common and psychological disorders such as post-traumatic stress disorder (PTSD) anxiety, depression, and substance abuse affect more than half of amputees in the longer term (33). However, only a small proportion of traumatic amputees access mental health care, possibly due to the associated stigma (1). Early counselling and psychological support should begin as soon after resuscitation as possible. PTSD is often overlooked, possibly because avoidance is a symptom of the disorder, and screening for mental health problems should be an important aspect of rehabilitation.

Amputation revision

Residual limb pain due to bone and soft tissue problems is nearly twice as common after a traumatic amputation than after amputation for non-traumatic indications (34). Common causes include heterotopic ossification, sharp bone ends, symptomatic neuromata, lack of end-bearing soft tissue padding via a secure myodesis, excess soft tissues, and poor-quality soft tissues in weight-bearing areas causing recurrent skin problems. Revision amputation should be considered when non-operative measures fail. A retrospective review of 71 revision cases reported improvement in 66% of confirmed neuromas, over 80% of patients with bone pathology, and 70% of patients with soft tissue problems (35).

Rehabilitation

The importance of rehabilitation in delivering good functional outcomes is evidenced by the startling results of the Military Extremity Trauma Amputation/Limb Salvage (METALS) study (24). Unlike the LEAP study, which found similar outcomes in civilians treated by amputation or limb salvage (36), military personnel undergoing amputation had significantly improved functional outcomes compared with those treated with limb salvage. Furthermore, unilateral and bilateral amputees were nearly three times more likely to be engaged in a vigorous sports or recreational activity than limb salvage patients and were less likely to screen positive for post-traumatic stress. The researchers suggested that the results might be explained by the focused rehabilitation military amputees receive early in their recovery and the ready access to optimal prostheses and robust reintegration programmes. In addition, military amputees are generally young and fit and may also have greater access to peer and external support early in their recovery, which may result in better outcomes. The benefit of a comprehensive extremity rehabilitation programme was also demonstrated in a series of limb salvage patients with severe traumatic lower extremity deficits (37).

Conclusion

Surgical advances have provided the means to reconstruct injuries that would have been previously amenable only to amputation. However, the surgeon's desire for reconstruction and the patient's wish for limb salvage must be balanced by the poor results of failed limb salvage and the good outcomes of successful amputation. An understanding of the therapeutic variables that affect outcome after both limb salvage and limb amputation will provide a platform for informed decision-making and will maximise the likelihood of a successful outcome.

References

1. **Perkins ZB, De'Ath HD, Sharp G, Tai NR.** Factors affecting outcome after traumatic limb amputation. Br J Surg. 2012;**99**(S1):75–86.
2. **McKenzie EJ, Bosse MJ, Kellam JF, Burgess AR, Webb LX, Swiontkowski MF,** et al. Factors influencing the decision to amputate or reconstruct after high-energy lower extremity trauma. J Trauma Acute Care Surg. 2002;**52**(4):641–9.

3. **National Clinical Guideline Centre (UK).** *Fractures (Complex): Assessment and Management.* London: National Institute for Health and Care Excellence (UK); 2016 Feb. NG37. https://www.nice.org.uk/guidance/ng37/chapter/Recommendations#hospital-settings

4. **Saddawi-Konefka D, Kim HM, Chung KC.** A systematic review of outcomes and complications of reconstruction and amputation for type IIIB and IIIC fractures of the tibia. Plast Reconstr Surg. 2008;**122**):1796–805.

5. **Bosse MJ, MacKenzie EJ, Kellam JF, Burgess AR, Webb LX, Swiontkowski MF, et al.** An analysis of outcomes of reconstruction or amputation after leg-threatening injuries. N Engl J Med. 2002;**347**(24):1924–31.

6. **Penn-Barwell JG.** Outcomes in lower limb amputation following trauma: a systematic review and meta-analysis. Injury. 2011;**42**(12):1474–9.

7. **Blair JA, Eisenstein ED, Pierrie SN, Gordon W, Owens JG, Hsu JR.** Lower extremity limb salvage: lessons learned from 14 years at war. J Orthop Trauma. 2016;**30**(Suppl 3):S11–S15.

8. **Caudle RJ, Stern PJ.** Severe open fractures of the tibia. J Bone Joint Surg Am. 1987;**69**(6):801–7.

9. **British Orthopaedic Association.** BOAST—Open fractures. London: BOA; December 2017. https://www.boa.ac.uk/standards-guidance/boasts.html

10. **Tintle SM, Keeling JJ, Shawen SB, Forsberg JA, Potter BK.** Traumatic and trauma-related amputations: part I: general principles and lower-extremity amputations. J Bone Joint Surg Am. 2010;**92**(17):2852–68.

11. **Perkins ZB, Yet B, Glasgow S, Cole E, Marsh W, Brohi K, et al.** Meta-analysis of prognostic factors for amputation following surgical repair of lower extremity vascular trauma. Br J Surg. 2015;**102**(5):436–50.

12. **Khalil IM, Livingston DH.** Intravascular shunts in complex lower limb trauma. J Vasc Surg. 1986;**4**(6):582–7.

13. **Bosse MJ, McCarthy ML, Jones AL, Webb LX, Sims SH, Sanders RW, et al.** The insensate foot following severe lower extremity trauma: an indication for amputation? J Bone Joint Surg Am. 2005;**87**(12):2601–8.

14. **Myerson MS, McGarvey WC, Henderson MR, Hakim J.** Morbidity after crush injuries to the foot. J Orthop Trauma. 1994;**8**(4):343–9.

15. **Turchin DC, Schemitsch EH, McKee MD, Waddell JP.** Do foot injuries significantly affect the functional outcome of multiply injured patients? J Orthop Trauma. 1999;**13**(1):1–4.

16. **Tran T, Thordarson D.** Functional outcome of multiply injured patients with associated foot injury. Foot Ankle Int. 2002;**23**(4):340–3.

17. **Castillo RC, Bosse MJ, MacKenzie EJ, Patterson BM, LEAP Study Group.** Impact of smoking on fracture healing and risk of complications in limb-threatening open tibia fractures. J Orthop Trauma. 2005;**19**(3):151–7.

18. **Scolaro JA, Schenker ML, Yannascoli S, Baldwin K, Mehta S, Ahn J.** Cigarette smoking increases complications following fracture: a systematic review. J Bone Joint Surg Am. 2014;**96**(8):674–81.

19. **Pluvy I, Panouillères M, Garrido I, Pauchot J, Saboye J, Chavoin JP, et al.** Smoking and plastic surgery, part II. Clinical implications: a systematic review with meta-analysis. Ann Chir Plast Esthet. 2015;**60**(1):e15–49.

20. **Sorensen LT.** Wound healing and infection in surgery. The clinical impact of smoking and smoking cessation: a systematic review and meta-analysis. Arch Surg. 2012;**147**(4):373–83.

21. **Gordon WT, O'Brien FP, Strauss JE, Andersen RC, Potter BK.** Outcomes associated with the internal fixation of long-bone fractures proximal to traumatic amputations. J Bone Joint Surg Am. 2010;**92**(13):2312–18.

22. **Tintle SM, LeBrun C, Ficke JR, Potter BK.** What is new in trauma-related amputations. J Orthop Trauma. 2016;**30**(Suppl 3):S16–S20.

23. **Wolthuis AM, Whitehead E, Ridler BM, Cowan AR, Campbell WB, Thompson JF.** Use of a pneumatic tourniquet improves outcome following trans-tibial amputation. Eur J Vasc Endovasc Surg. 2006;**31**(6):642–5.

24. **Doukas WC, Hayda RA, Frisch HM, Andersen RC, Mazurek MT, Ficke JR,** et al. The Military Extremity Trauma Amputation/Limb Salvage (METALS) Study: outcomes of amputation versus limb salvage following major lower-extremity trauma. J Bone Joint Surg Am. 2013;**95**(2):138–45.

25. **Ghali S, Harris PA, Khan U, Pearse M, Nanchahal J.** Leg length preservation with pedicled fillet of foot flaps after traumatic amputations. Plast Reconstr Surg. 2005;**115**(2):498–505.

26. **Albino FP, Seidel R, Brown BJ, Crone CG, Attinger CE.** Through knee amputation: technique modifications and surgical outcomes. Arch Plast Surg. 2014;**41**(5):562–70.

27. **Taylor BC, Poka A, French BG, Fowler TT, Mehta S.** Gritti-Stokes amputations in the trauma patient: clinical comparisons and subjective outcomes. J Bone Joint Surg Am. 2012;**94**(7):602–8.

28. **Harris AM, Althausen PL, Kellam J, Bosse MJ, Castillo R, Lower Extremity Assessment Project (LEAP) Study Group.** Complications following limb-threatening lower extremity trauma. J Orthop Trauma. 2009;**23**(1):1–6.

29. **Jain A, Glass GE, Ahmadi H, Mackey S, Simmons J, Hettiaratchy S, Pearse MF, Nanchahal J.** Delayed amputation following trauma increases residual lower limb infection. J Plast Reconstr Aesthet Surg. 2013;**66**(4):531–7.

30. **Glass GE, Barrett SP, Sanderson F, Pearse MF, Nanchahal J.** The microbiological basis for a revised antibiotic regimen in high-energy tibial fractures: preventing deep infections by nosocomial organisms. J Plast Reconstr Aesthet Surg. 2011;**64**(3):375–80.

31. **Castillo RC, MacKenzie EJ, Wegener ST, Bosse MJ, LEAP Study Group.** Prevalence of chronic pain seven years following limb threatening lower extremity trauma. Pain. 2006;**124**(3):321–9.

32. **Flor H.** Phantom-limb pain: characteristics, causes, and treatment. Lancet Neurol. 2002;**1**(3):182–9.

33. **McCarthy ML, MacKenzie EJ, Edwin D, Bosse MJ, Castillo RC, Starr A,** et al. Psychological distress associated with severe lower-limb injury. J Bone Joint Surg Am. 2003;**85**-a(9):1689–97.

34. **Ephraim PL, Wegener ST, MacKenzie EJ, Dillingham TR, Pezzin LE.** Phantom pain, residual limb pain, and back pain in amputees: results of a national survey. Arch Physical Med Rehab. 2005;**86**(10):1910–19.

35. **Bourke HE, Yelden KC, Robinson KP, Sooriakumaran S, Ward DA.** Is revision surgery following lower-limb amputation a worthwhile procedure? A retrospective review of 71 cases. Injury. 2011;**42**(7):660–6.

36. **Busse JW, Jacobs CL, Swiontkowski MF, Bosse MJ, Bhandari M, Evidence-Based Orthopaedic Trauma Working Group.** Complex limb salvage or early amputation for severe lower-limb injury: a meta-analysis of observational studies. J Orthop Trauma. 2007;**21**(1):70–6.

37. **Bedigrew KM, Patzkowski JC, Wilken JM, Owens JG, Blanck RV, Stinner DJ, et al.** Can an integrated orthotic and rehabilitation program decrease pain and improve function after lower extremity trauma? Clin Orthop Relat Res. 2014;**472**(10):3017–25.

Chapter 13

Infection

Summary

1. Infection is the commonest major complication after open trauma and a high level of clinical suspicion is key for early diagnosis.

2. A multidisciplinary approach is mandatory, including orthopaedic and plastic surgeons, microbiology and infectious disease consultants, and radiologists.

3. Evaluation of both local and systemic host factors that predispose to infection, are essential before commencing treatment.

4. Diagnostic work-up commences ideally after stopping antibiotics in stable patients and includes blood cultures if febrile, X-rays for implant loosening and bone changes, ultrasound-guided aspiration, and/or deep tissue sampling. Microbiological diagnosis may be difficult using traditional techniques and culture-negative cases should be treated proactively by a dedicated multidisciplinary team (MDT).

5. Cornerstones of effective treatment are the prompt removal of sessile bacteria within the biofilm by aggressive wound excision and the elimination of planktonic bacteria by targeted, culture-specific antimicrobial chemotherapy.

6. Removal of internal fixation devices is usually required except in early infection due to low-virulence organisms. Treatment by implant retention and antibiotic suppression should be part of a clear MDT plan and failure of treatment demands reevaluation.

Introduction

Infection is the most feared and challenging complication in the treatment of open tibial fractures. Microorganisms can adhere as a biofilm on the surface of damaged bone, necrotic tissue, and internal fixation devices, and become resistant to phagocytosis and most antimicrobial agents (1). Established infection can delay healing and recovery, cause permanent functional loss, and potentially lead to amputation of the affected limb. The incidence of infection after severe open tibial fractures was reported to be over 30% in the 1980s and 1990s (2, 3). Although there is evidence of a possible reduction in incidence in the past decade (4), the Lower Extremity Assessment Project (LEAP) study has shown that severe lower extremity trauma continues to be associated with infective complications necessitating additional operative treatment in a significant number of cases (5). Furthermore, greater bacterial virulence and increasing age and associated co-morbidities of the fracture population ensure that infection after open trauma remains a challenge.

Definition and classification

There are no agreed criteria for diagnosing fracture infection (3, 6). The Centers for Disease Control (CDC) guidelines for surgical site infection (SSI) are often quoted but the complexity of an infected fracture is not covered by these guidelines (3, 7). Although comprehensive definitions are lacking, there is an accepted classification of infection after trauma according to the time of onset, which reflects the extent of biofilm formation and fracture-healing status, with implications for treatment (3, 8).

1. Early infections (less than 2 weeks) are easily diagnosed clinically since the classic signs of infection (swelling, redness, pain) are usually present in addition to delayed wound healing and drainage, haematoma, and accompanying pyrexia. Virulent organisms, like *Staphylococcus aureus* are common pathogens and an immature biofilm may be present (9). Osteomyelitis and accompanying inflammation and osteolysis will not have developed and fracture instability is unlikely at this early stage (3).

2. Delayed infections (2–10 weeks) may be associated with signs consistent with either early or late infection but infections are typically due to less virulent organisms, such as *Staphylococcus epidermidis* (9). The biofilm is more mature and relatively resistant to antibiotic therapy and host defences. In addition, bacterial bone invasion and osteomyelitis will be more advanced, with implications for fracture healing and stability (10, 11).

3. Late-onset infections (more than 10 weeks) are characterised by subtle signs of infection, without systemic manifestation, and are usually caused by low-virulence organisms (9). Fracture healing may be complete or incomplete but chronic inflammation (osteomyelitis) causes local tissue damage and osteolysis potentially leading to fixation instability, with implications for the residual hardware. Periosteal new bone produces an involucrum in response to the persistent low-grade inflammation caused by the infection and these changes often necessitate extensive and repeated wound excision, resulting in bone- and soft tissue defects (12).

Diagnosis

Acute cases should be carefully monitored and local signs of infection must be considered diagnostic, even in the presence of negative cultures. Delayed wound healing and drainage or an active sinus are definitive signs of infection. Persistent elevation or a secondary rise in C-reactive protein is a useful indicator of infection (13). Plain radiology findings are usually normal in early infection and callus formation and the presence of hardware may mask the later subtle radiological features of infection (14). Whilst serial radiographs are useful to assess fracture healing and implant stability, computed tomography (CT) provides more bone architecture detail as well as signs of implant loosening (3). Markers for active infection such as cortical reaction, sequestra, sinuses, and abscess formation in the adjacent soft tissue may also be evident on CT scans (15). Whilst magnetic resonance imaging (MRI) is useful to evaluate soft tissue involvement and intramedullary infection, metal artefacts, bone oedema, and scarring may mimic infection and impair correct evaluation (16).

Nuclear imaging modalities are sensitive but not specific, especially when underlying bone abnormalities are present and discrimination between infection and post-traumatic bone formation is difficult (3, 17). Hybrid imaging (single-photon emission computed tomography (SPECT)/CT) can localise the suspected infection and facilitate the discrimination between bone- and soft tissue infection. Sensitivities over 95% and specificities from 75–99% have been reported in acute and subacute bone- and soft tissue infection (17).

Microbiology

Pathogens present in open wounds tend to evolve from initial contamination with multiple low-virulence pathogens to early infections including nosocomial organisms, which may be multi-drug resistant, through to mature infections caused by *Staphylococci* (18). Infection is usually due to metabolically quiescent bacteria growing in protected biofilms on the metal implants and in necrotic bone, which makes the pathogens difficult to identify using traditional culture techniques (19). At least three tissue biopsies should be taken in regions of perceived infection such as necrotic bone tissue or non-unions and around the implant (9). Bone biopsies are the diagnostic gold standard, particularly in delayed and chronic infection (20). If the same microorganism is cultured from at least two separate biopsies, it is probably relevant. A single positive biopsy of a virulent species such as *S. aureus* or *Escherichia coli* may also represent an infection. Antibiotics should be stopped for at least 2 weeks before sampling to avoid transforming bacterial species into viable but non-culturable forms when the cultures may become falsely negative (21, 22). Extended culture for up to

Box 13.1 Risk factors for infection

severe soft tissue damage

associated vascular trauma

extensive bone loss

delayed presentation:

♦ late antibiotic prophylaxis (beyond 1 hour of injury)

♦ late soft tissue cover (beyond 3 days)

compromised host physiology

♦ diabetes

♦ smoking

14 days of incubation may identify difficult-to-culture pathogens, but interpretation of extended culture results must be correlated with the clinical picture (23). Patients with clear clinical signs of infection but negative cultures should be treated as infected (24).

Other techniques to improve the yield of positive cultures, especially after pre-treatment with antibiotics, include sonication of removed hardware and molecular methods using polymerase chain reaction (PCR) (25, 26).

Host evaluation

An evaluation of the local and systemic host risk factors is essential before considering treatment (Box 13.1). High-risk local factors include severe soft tissue and bone damage and compromised local vascularity. Systemic factors include a previous history of infection and compromised physiology including smoking, diabetes, peripheral vascular disease, alcoholism, and polytrauma (12). Infection with virulent organisms in a patient with local and systemic risk factors may preclude complex reconstructive procedures, and limited non-ablative surgery with antibiotic suppression or amputation should be considered (27).

Repatriation

Aeromedical evacuation of both civilian and military trauma victims by long-distance air flight is increasingly common. Recent studies of inter-hospital transfers of trauma victims have highlighted frequent wound contamination with highly resistant bacteria, particularly in patients nursed in an intensive care setting (28). Resistant organisms associated with inter-country transfer include multi-resistant *Acinetobacter* spp. and *Klebsiella pneumoniae*, methicillin-resistant *S. aureus* (MRSA), vancomycin-resistant *Enterococci*, and multi-resistant *Clostridium difficile* (29). Sound infection prevention strategies are essential to prevent dissemination of multi-resistant organisms from patients who have been admitted to hospitals in other countries. In addition, clinicians may also need to individualise empiric antibiotic prescribing patterns to reflect the risk of multi-resistant organisms in transferred patients.

Treatment

The principles of treatment include the removal of sessile (anchored) bacteria within the biofilm by wound excision and the elimination of planktonic (free-floating) bacteria by targeted antimicrobial chemotherapy. An effective wound excision combined with high-dose antibiotics achieves a rapid reduction in the bacterial load (3). An MDT approach is essential to address the fracture and soft tissue components, identify the pathogens, and deliver effective antimicrobial therapy whilst optimising the health of the host (30).

Wound excision combined with copious low-pressure saline lavage is a cornerstone of treatment, and radical excision of necrotic and infected tissue, both bone and soft tissue, may be required. Wound excision should not be limited by concerns of creating a bone or soft tissue defect because failing to excise compromised tissues may leave viable bacterial behind within the biofilm, which will lead to recurrence of the disease (31, 32). Multiple tissue samples from different surgical sites should be obtained using sterile instruments. Haematomas must be drained as they are an excellent growth medium for bacteria (9). The index operation should also include an evaluation of fracture stability with removal of unstable fixation and revision fixation as required (Box 13.2). An adequate soft tissue envelope is essential and flap cover may

Box 13.2 Indications for fixation revision

fracture instability
intramedullary fixation
compromised soft tissues
poor host physiology
virulent/resistant pathogens

be necessary. Alternatively, negative pressure dressings are employed between serial wound excision prior to definitive soft tissue cover.

Antimicrobial therapy

Initial intravenous broad-spectrum therapy is started after multiple microbial samples have been obtained at wound excision and continued until the pathogens and their sensitivities are identified. The duration of intravenous therapy depends on pathogen virulence and antibiotic sensitivities, as well as the initial host response to treatment. Patients with clinically infected wounds but negative cultures should be treated aggressively with empirical coverage for Gram positive and Gram negative microbes, including MRSA (24).

After a minimum of 2 weeks' intravenous therapy, a switch to oral therapy with good bioavailability can be considered (33, 34).

If the hardware is retained, the aim of antibiotic therapy is suppression of the infection until the fracture has healed and the hardware can be removed (9). However, curative treatment with implant retention is only effective with a biofilm-active antibiotic, such as rifampicin against *Staphylococci* and quinolones against Gram negative organisms (Box 13.2) (35–37). Rifampicin must be combined with a second antibiotic to prevent the development of resistance. Quinolones such as ciprofloxacin or levofloxacin are effective oral partners to rifampicin against *Staphylococci* (38). Bacteria resistant to biofilm-active antibiotics will not be eradicated if the internal fixation is retained and hardware removal is strongly recommended (1, 3).

Application of antimicrobials at the site of infection can achieve high local antibiotic concentrations, which may be useful in cases with impaired vascularity and as an aid for dead-space management (3). Common carries include non-resorbable polymethylmethacrylate (PMMA) and resorbable materials such as calcium sulfate. However, there is no clear evidence for the addition of local antibiotics to systemic therapy. In addition, colonisation of bone cement, particularly after antibiotics have been eluted, may promote ongoing infection or even induce antibiotic resistance (39) and calcium sulfate preparations may be associated with chronic wound discharge (3).

Early infection

Hardware colonisation and biofilm formation are relatively immature (40, 41) and retention of the fixation device may be considered as wound excision will reduce the bacterial load and may clear an immature biofilm and systemic antibiotics will treat the remainder of the infection. However a number of prerequisites must be fulfilled (Box 13.2). Effective wound excision and irrigation must be performed, which may not be possible with intramedullary fixation.

In addition, the fixation must be stable, advanced signs of established infection should not present, and the infecting organisms must be sensitive to antibiotics (42). A 12-week course of antibiotics is recommended with retained implants or up to 6 weeks after implant removal (9, 43). Once the fracture has healed, implant removal is recommended to reduce the risk of recurrent infection (44).

Delayed infection

The biofilm is more mature and osteomyelitis is becoming increasingly established and the surgical decision-making should tend towards radical wound excision and implant revision, particularly if there has been a delay in diagnosis and treatment or if infection has recurred after initial therapy. In a study of patients who developed infection within 6 weeks of fracture fixation treated with wound excision, antibiotics, and hardware retention, fracture healing was achieved in only 71% of the patients. In addition, open fractures and intramedullary fixation were predictors for treatment failure (45). In a similar study of infections within 16 weeks of fixation, successful union was reported in 68%, although 38% of patients with successful bone healing required hardware removed for persistent infection after union and only 49% of the original study group achieved healing and were free of infection after 6 months (44).

Late infection

Inflammation and osteolysis are usually evident in infections developing after 10 weeks and instability of the fracture fixation is often present, resulting in delayed or non-union (3). In addition, involucra and fibrous tissue in the infected area act as a barrier around necrotic bone necessitating an extensive wound excision with possible creation of bone- and soft tissue defects. Preoperative imaging studies are helpful to assess the extent of fracture healing and to plan the resection margins but staged procedures are commonly required. Antibiotic spacers may be useful adjuncts for dead-space management and local antibiotic delivery. Hardware removal is mandatory but bone stability must be preserved and external fixation can be a temporary or definitive solution.

Cases of longstanding therapy-resistant non-unions should be considered infected until proven otherwise (46) and molecular diagnostics are recommended if traditional cultures are negative (47).

References

1. **Zimmerli W, Trampuz A, Ochsner PE.** Prosthetic-joint infections. N Engl J Med. 2004;351(16):1645–54.
2. **Patzakis MJ, Wilkins J.** Factors influencing infection rate in open fracture wounds. Clin Orthop Rel Res. 1989;243(0009-921X (Print)):36–40.

3. **Metsemakers WJ, Kuehl R, Moriarty TF, Richards RG, Verhofstad MHJ, Borens O,** et al. Infection after fracture fixation: current surgical and microbiological concepts. Injury. 2016;49:511–22.

4. **Ktistakis I, Giannoudi M, Giannoudis PV.** Infection rates after open tibial fractures: are they decreasing? Injury. 2014;45(7):1025–7.

5. **Harris AM, Althausen PL, Kellam J, Bosse MJ, Castillo R, Lower Extremity Assessment Project (LEAP) Study Group,** et al. Complications following limb-threatening lower extremity trauma. J Orthop Trauma. 2009;23(1):1–6.

6. **Cook GE, Markel DC, Ren W, Webb LX, McKee MD, Schemitsch EH.** Infection in orthopaedics. J Orthop Trauma. 2015;29(Suppl 12):S19–23.

7. **Mangram AJ, Horan TC, Pearson ML, Silver LC, Jarvis WR.** Guideline for Prevention of Surgical Site Infection, 1999. Centers for Disease Control and Prevention (CDC) Hospital Infection Control Practices Advisory Committee. Am J Infect Control. 1999;27(2):97–132; quiz 133–4; discussion 96.

8. **Willenegger H, Roth B.** [Treatment tactics and late results in early infection following osteosynthesis]. Unfallchirurgie. 1986;12(5):241–6.

9. **Trampuz A, Zimmerli W.** Diagnosis and treatment of infections associated with fracture-fixation devices. Injury. 2006;37(Suppl 2):S59–66.

10. **Lovati AB, Romanò CL, Bottagisio M, Monti L, De Vecchi E, Previdi S,** et al. Modeling *Staphylococcus epidermidis*-induced non-unions: subclinical and clinical evidence in rats. PLoS One. 2016;11(1):e0147447.

11. **Bilgili F, Balci HI, Karaytug K, Sariyilmaz K, Atalar AC, Bozdag E,** et al. Can normal fracture healing be achieved when the implant is retained on the basis of infection? An experimental animal model. Clin Orthop Relat Res. 2015;473(10):3190–6.

12. **Willey M, Karam M.** Impact of infection on fracture fixation. Orthop Clin North Am. 2016;47(2):357–64.

13. **Neumaier M, Scherer MA.** C-reactive protein levels for early detection of postoperative infection after fracture surgery in 787 patients. Acta Orthop. 2008;79(3):428–32.

14. **Wheat J.** Diagnostic strategies in osteomyelitis. Am J Med. 1985;78(6b):218–24.

15. **Gross T, Kaim AH, Regazzoni P, Widmer AF.** Current concepts in posttraumatic osteomyelitis: a diagnostic challenge with new imaging options. J Trauma. 2002;52(6):1210–19.

16. **Ledermann HP, Kaim A, Bongartz G, Steinbrich W.** Pitfalls and limitations of magnetic resonance imaging in chronic posttraumatic osteomyelitis. Eur Radiol. 2000;10(11):1815–23.

17. **Love C, Palestro CJ.** Nuclear medicine imaging of bone infections. Clin Radiol. 2016;71(7):632–46.

18. **Yun HC, Murray CK, Nelson KJ, Bosse MJ.** Infection after orthopaedic trauma: prevention and treatment. J Orthop Trauma. 2016;30(Suppl 3):S21–6.

19. **Costerton JW, Post JC, Ehrlich GD, Hu FZ, Kreft R, Nistico L,** et al. New methods for the detection of orthopedic and other biofilm infections. FEMS Immunol Med Microbiol. 2011;61(2):133–40.

20. **Zuluaga AF, Galvis W, Jaimes F, Vesga O.** Lack of microbiological concordance between bone and non-bone specimens in chronic osteomyelitis: an observational study. BMC Infect Dis. 2002;2:8.

21. **Pasquaroli S, Zandri G, Vignaroli C, Vuotto C, Donelli G, Biavasco F.** Antibiotic pressure can induce the viable but non-culturable state in *Staphylococcus aureus* growing in biofilms. J Antimicrob Chemother. 2013;**68**(8):1812–17.

22. **Malekzadeh D, Osmon DR, Lahr BD, Hanssen AD, Berbari EF.** Prior use of antimicrobial therapy is a risk factor for culture-negative prosthetic joint infection. Clin Orthop Relat Res. 2010;**468**(8):2039–45.

23. **Schwotzer N, Wahl P, Fracheboud D, Gautier E, Chuard C.** Optimal culture incubation time in orthopedic device-associated infections: a retrospective analysis of prolonged 14-day incubation. J Clin Microbiol. 2014;**52**(1):61–6.

24. **Gitajn IL, Heng M, Weaver MJ, Ehrlichman LK, Harris MB.** Culture-negative infection after operative fixation of fractures. J Orthop Trauma. 2016;**30**(10):538–44.

25. **Yano MH, Klautau GB, da Silva CB, Nigro S, Avanzi O, Mercadante MT,** et al. Improved diagnosis of infection associated with osteosynthesis by use of sonication of fracture fixation implants. J Clin Microbiol. 2014;**52**(12):4176–82.

26. **Greenwood-Quaintance KE, Uhl JR, Hanssen AD, Sampath R, Mandrekar JN, Patel R.** Diagnosis of prosthetic joint infection by use of PCR-electrospray ionization mass spectrometry. J Clin Microbiol. 2014;**52**(2):642–9.

27. **Cierny G, 3rd, Mader JT, Penninck JJ.** A clinical staging system for adult osteomyelitis. Clin Orthop Relat Res. 2003(414):7–24.

28. **Maegele M, Gregor S, Steinhausen E, Bouillon B, Heiss MM, Perbix W, Wappler F,** et al. The long-distance tertiary air transfer and care of tsunami victims: injury pattern and microbiological and psychological aspects. Crit Care Med. 2005;**33**(5):1136–40.

29. **Rogers BA, Aminzadeh Z, Hayashi Y, Paterson DL.** Country-to-country transfer of patients and the risk of multi-resistant bacterial infection. Clin Infect Dis. 2011;**53**(1):49–56.

30. **Ziran BH, Rao N, Hall RA.** A dedicated team approach enhances outcomes of osteomyelitis treatment. Clin Orthop Relat Res. 2003(414):31–6.

31. **Patzakis MJ, Zalavras CG.** Chronic posttraumatic osteomyelitis and infected nonunion of the tibia: current management concepts. J Am Acad Orthop Surg. 2005;**13**(6):417–27.

32. **Simpson AH, Deakin M, Latham JM.** Chronic osteomyelitis. The effect of the extent of surgical resection on infection-free survival. J Bone Joint Surg Br. 2001;**83**(3):403–7.

33. **Daver NG, Shelburne SA, Atmar RL, Giordano TP, Stager CE, Reitman CA** et al. Oral step-down therapy is comparable to intravenous therapy for *Staphylococcus aureus* osteomyelitis. J Infect. 2007;**54**(6):539–44.

34. **Spellberg B, Lipsky BA.** Systemic antibiotic therapy for chronic osteomyelitis in adults. Clin Infect Dis. 2012;**54**(3):393–407.

35. **Widmer AF, Gaechter A, Ochsner PE, Zimmerli W.** Antimicrobial treatment of orthopedic implant-related infections with rifampin combinations. Clin Infect Dis. 1992;**14**(6):1251–3.

36. **Zimmerli W, Widmer AF, Blatter M, Frei R, Ochsner PE.** Role of rifampin for treatment of orthopedic implant-related staphylococcal infections: a randomized controlled trial. Foreign-Body Infection (FBI) Study Group. Jama. 1998;**279**(19):1537–41.

37. **Aboltins CA, Dowsey MM, Buising KL, Peel TN, Daffy JR, Choong PF,** et al. Gram-negative prosthetic joint infection treated with debridement, prosthesis

retention and antibiotic regimens including a fluoroquinolone. Clin Microbiol Infect. 2011;17(6):862–7.

38. Senneville E, Joulie D, Legout L, Valette M, Dezèque H, Beltrand E, et al. Outcome and predictors of treatment failure in total hip/knee prosthetic joint infections due to *Staphylococcus aureus*. Clin Infect Dis. 2011;53(4):334–40.

39. Hake ME, Young H, Hak DJ, Stahel PF, Hammerberg EM, Mauffrey C. Local antibiotic therapy strategies in orthopaedic trauma: Practical tips and tricks and review of the literature. Injury. 2015;46(8):1447–56.

40. Costerton JW. Biofilm theory can guide the treatment of device-related orthopaedic infections. Clin Orthop Relat Res. 2005(437):7–11.

41. Nishitani K, Sutipornpalangkul W, de Mesy Bentley KL, Varrone JJ, Bello-Irizarry SN, Ito H, et al. Quantifying the natural history of biofilm formation in vivo during the establishment of chronic implant-associated *Staphylococcus aureus* osteomyelitis in mice to identify critical pathogen and host factors. J Orthop Res. 2015;33(9):1311–19.

42. Merritt K, Dowd JD. Role of internal fixation in infection of open fractures: studies with *Staphylococcus aureus* and *Proteus mirabilis*. J Orthop Res. 1987;5(1):23–8.

43. Trebse R, Pisot V, Trampuz A. Treatment of infected retained implants. J Bone Joint Surg Br. 2005;87(2):249–56.

44. Rightmire E, Zurakowski D, Vrahas M. Acute infections after fracture repair: management with hardware in place. Clin Orthop Relat Res. 2008;466(2):466–72.

45. Berkes M, Obremskey WT, Scannell B, Ellington JK, Hymes RA, Bosse M, et al. Maintenance of hardware after early postoperative infection following fracture internal fixation. J Bone Joint Surg Am. 2010;92(4):823–8.

46. Tsang ST, Mills LA, Frantzias J, Baren JP, Keating JF, Simpson AH. Exchange nailing for nonunion of diaphyseal fractures of the tibia: our results and an analysis of the risk factors for failure. Bone Joint J. 2016;98-b(4):534–41.

47. Palmer MP, Altman DT, Altman GT, Sewecke JJ, Ehrlich GD, Hu FZ, et al., Can we trust intraoperative culture results in nonunions? J Orthop Trauma. 2014;28(7):384–90.

Chapter 14

Open Tibial Fractures in Children

Summary

1. The initial management of a child's open fracture is the same as is recommended for adults. There is no evidence children have greater resistance to infection once the barrier of soft tissue cover of the fracture has been compromised by injury.

2. The soft tissues of children do not have a greater regenerative potential and soft tissue reconstruction techniques involve the same strategies as in adults.

3. Fracture fixation will need to consider the presence of physes. Flexible intramedullary nails, Kirschner wires, plates introduced by minimally invasive methods, and external fixators have their indications.

4. Bone loss in very young children (under 6 years) may be managed expectantly if the defect is small as spontaneous periosteal bone formation may occur. In older children, bone replacement by autografts or bone regeneration methods is required.

5. Skeletal injuries in children older than 12 years behave as in adults and have higher complication rates. Delayed or non-unions will require a more active treatment strategy.

Timing of wound excision after injury

An early publication reported a halving of infection rates in children with open fractures if debrided within 6 hours of injury (1). This was contested by a multicentre review of 554 open paediatric fractures where there was no significant difference in the incidence of infection when wound excision was performed on either side of the 6-hour threshold (2). A recent publication from the UK that reported compliance with the last issue of Standards of Treatment (British Orthopaedic Association/British Association of Plastic, Reconstructive and Aesthetic Surgeons (BOA/BAPRAS)) in 2009 had antibiotics given intravenously on arrival in the emergency department and had all injuries debrided on the day of admission or the next day if the patient arrived after midnight. The injuries were managed jointly by orthopaedic and plastic surgery consultants.

The incidence of deep infection was reported at 4.9%, which is—considering that 70% of the 61 open tibial fractures were of Gustilo–Anderson grade 3—commendably low (3). We recommend antibiotics are given within 1 hour of injury and the timing of wound excision for high-energy open fractures (presumed Gustilo–Anderson grade III) in children and adults is the same: immediately for those compromised by compartment syndrome, ischaemia of the limb, heavy contamination, or as part of a multiple injury, and within 12 hours if a solitary injury.

Skeletal stabilisation

Reports of low-grade Gustilo–Anderson open fractures being treated successfully by superficial wound excision and irrigation with antibiotics and cast stabilisation are misleading (4). These reports are a heterogeneous mix of open injuries with, in one report, tibial fractures constituting only 4% of the injuries (5). Non-operative management of open tibial fractures in children remains contentious and potentially dangerous (6).

Flexible intramedullary nails, plate and screws, Kirschner wires, and external fixators have proponents for use in fracture stabilisation. With flexible intramedullary nails, choosing the suitable injury type is important; stability depends on an intact soft tissue envelope and these nails are less effective for stabilisation in children over 50 kg weight (7). For those injury patterns and patients where this method is considered suitable, immediate flexible nailing and primary wound closure is associated with a low rate of complications. Classic plate fixation may appear to be linked to higher infection although it is unclear in the report admonishing this method of stabilisation if the injuries were significantly contaminated or if definitive soft tissue cover was accomplished at the same time as fixation (3). Use of plates in a minimally invasive manner on the lateral side of the tibia may be best suited to the less severe types of open injury (8).

External fixation may be used as a temporary stabilisation device or definitively. Monolateral and circular devices have their roles. Tensioned wires with circular fixators are able to capture short metaphyseal segments well, whereas monolateral devices based on half-pins are easier to apply for most surgeons. Circular fixators can also be used for reconstruction when managing bone defects (9–11).

The choice of definitive skeletal stabilisation will depend on the fracture location and pattern, the degree of comminution or bone loss, contamination, and the availability of definitive soft tissue cover. In the event that definitive stabilisation and soft tissue cover cannot be performed at the time of initial wound excision, we recommend temporary spanning external fixation is used in conjunction with temporary dressings. In fractures contaminated heavily at the time of injury, definitive external fixation is recommended.

Soft tissue reconstruction

Several studies have confirmed early definitive soft tissue cover is as necessary for children as it is for adults (3, 9, 12–15). Delayed involvement of a plastic surgeon in management leads to more complications (14). The choice of cover will depend on the size and location of the defect, local tissue conditions, and the zone of injury. Split-thickness skin grafts, local fasciocutaneous, and free flaps are used. The overriding principles are the same as for adults and include: wound extension by incision; meticulous excision of contaminated and devitalised tissues; and early definitive cover (16). Grade 3B and 3C injuries are particularly challenging and demand the highest levels of input from all areas. A systematic review of free tissue transfer for open tibial fractures in children found that the commonest choice appears to be muscle flaps followed by perforator flaps. There is an increasing use of perforator flaps (e.g. anterolateral thigh flap) citing advantages of consistent anatomy, reduced donor site morbidity, and the supply of durable native skin that is ideal for the foot and ankle regions. The overall free flap failure rate for children's open tibial fractures is similar to that for adults at approximately 5% (12).

Bone reconstruction

Bone defects occur from loss at the scene of injury or after wound excision. The critical size of the defect that results in a non-union in children is unknown but it is recognised that young children can bridge defects from periosteal new bone formation in a manner that occurs rarely in adults (6). In very young children (possibly under 6 years) an expectant approach in the first 6 weeks after definitive stabilisation and wound closure may be taken if serial radiographs indicate increasing contributions of periosteal new bone formation across the defect, thereby avoiding further surgery (17). In older children, and certainly those over the age of 11 years (18), these defects should be managed by autologous bone grafts or through bone regeneration using distraction osteogenesis. The choice of technique will depend on the size of the defect, soft tissue envelope for bone grafting, availability of autogenous graft material, and familiarity of the surgeon with the techniques of bone transport or acute shortening across the defect and bone lengthening from an osteotomy at a different level (9, 19). Small defects of <3 cm where the underlying bone and covering soft tissue are amenable to further surgery may be treated simply with autologous bone graft harvested from the posterior iliac crest.

Union and infection

The objective in treating open fractures in children is the same as in adults—infection-free union. Healing in young children is different; fracture union times are shorter. However, there is evidence to suggest this advantage is lost by the age of 10–12 years and, especially with high-energy tibial fractures, there is an increasing likelihood for complications including non-union (3, 16, 17, 20, 21). Overall infection rates across the fracture types can vary between 3 and 8% (17, 18, 22). These figures may mislead as Gustilo–Anderson type I and II fractures are the most common and do not usually become infected. Infection rates are higher with Gustilo–Anderson type IIIB fractures and can reach 21% (23, 24). However, the combined orthoplastic approach as advocated here resulted in deep infection rates of less than 7% for type IIIB fractures in children (3).

Conclusion

There are greater similarities than differences when the treatment of open tibial fractures in children is compared with adults. The emphasis remains on early antibiotic administration, prompt and meticulous wound excision by orthopaedic and plastic surgery consultants, and early definitive soft tissue cover. It is important to note that children do not have an enhanced regenerative capacity in their soft tissues and, as in adults, all non-viable tissue should be excised. The techniques for soft tissue reconstruction in children are the same as with adults. The method of fracture stabilisation can vary depending on the fracture pattern and location, degree of contamination, presence of bone loss, and age of the child. Very young children may recover from bone loss spontaneously by periosteal new bone formation. Older children will require bone grafting or bone regeneration.

References

1. **Kreder HJ.** A review of open tibia fractures in children. J Ped Orthop. 1995;15(4):482.
2. **Skaggs D, Friend L, Alman B, Chambers H.** The effect of surgical delay on acute infection following 554 open fractures in children. J Bone Joint Surg. 2005;87(1):8–12.
3. **Nandra RS, Wu F, Gaffey A, Bache CE.** The management of open tibial fractures in children: a retrospective case series of eight years' experience of 61 cases at a paediatric specialist centre. Bone Joint J. 2017;99-b(4):544–53.
4. **Bazzi AA, Brooks JT, Jain A, Ain MC, Tis JE, Sponseller PD.** Is nonoperative treatment of pediatric type I open fractures safe and effective? J Child Orthop. 2014;8(6):467–71.
5. **Godfrey J, Choi PD, Shabtai L, Nossov SB, Williams A, Lindberg AW,** et al. Management of pediatric type i open fractures in the emergency department or

operating room: a multicenter perspective. J Pediatr Orthop. 2017. DOI:10.1097/BPO.0000000000000972.

6. **Stewart DG, Jr, Kay RM, Skaggs DL.** Open fractures in children. Principles of evaluation and management. J Bone Joint Surg Am. 2005;**87**(12):2784–98.

7. **Pandya NK.** Flexible intramedullary nailing of unstable and/or open tibia shaft fractures in the pediatric population. J Pediatr Orthop. 2016;**36**(Suppl 1):S19–23.

8. **Ozkul E, Gem M, Arslan H, Alemdar C, Azboy I, Arslan SG.** Minimally invasive plate osteosynthesis in open pediatric tibial fractures. J Pediatr Orthop. 2016;**36**(4):416–22.

9. **Laine JC, Cherkashin A, Samchukov M, Birch JG, Rathjen KE.** The management of soft tissue and bone loss in type iiib and iiic pediatric open tibia fractures. J Pediatr Orthop. 2016;**36**(5):453–8.

10. **Tafazal S, Madan SS, Ali F, Padman M, Swift S, Jones S,** et al. Management of paediatric tibial fractures using two types of circular external fixator: Taylor spatial frame and Ilizarov circular fixator. J Child Orthop. 2014;**8**(3):273–9.

11. **Monsell FP, Howells NR, Lawniczak D, Jeffcote B, Mitchell SR.** High-energy open tibial fractures in children: treatment with a programmable circular external fixator. J Bone Joint Surg Br. 2012;**94**(7):989–93.

12. **Jabir S, Sheikh F, Fitzgerald O'Connor E, Griffiths M, Niranjan N.** A systematic review of the applications of free tissue transfer for paediatric lower limb salvage following trauma. J Plast Surg Hand Surg. 2015;**49**(5):251–9.

13. **Choudry U, Moran S, Karacor Z.** Soft-tissue coverage and outcome of Gustilo grade IIIB midshaft tibia fractures: a 15-year experience. Plast Reconstr Surg. 2008;**122**(2):479–85.

14. **Rao P, Schaverien M, Stewart K.** Soft tissue management of children's open tibial fractures—a review of seventy children over twenty years. Ann R Coll Surg Engl. 2010;**92**(4):320–5.

15. **Stewart KJ, Tytherleigh-Strong G, Bharathwaj S, Quaba AA.** The soft tissue management of children's open tibial fractures. J R Coll Surg Edinb. 1999;**44**(1):24.

16. **Glass GE, Pearse M, Nanchahal J.** The ortho-plastic management of Gustilo grade IIIB fractures of the tibia in children: a systematic review of the literature. Injury. 2009;**40**(8):876–9.

17. **Grimard G, Naudie D, Laberge LC, Hamdy RC.** Open fractures of the tibia in children. Clin Orthop Relat Res. 1996;(332):62–70.

18. **Song KM, Sangeorzan B, Benirschke S, Browne R.** Open fractures of the tibia in children. J Pediatr Orthop. 1996;**16**(5):635–9.

19. **Arslan H, Ozkul E, Gem M, Alemdar C, Sahin I, Kisin B.** Segmental bone loss in pediatric lower extremity fractures: indications and results of bone transport. J Pediatr Orthop. 2015;**35**(2):e8–12.

20. **Gougoulias N, Khanna A, Maffulli N.** Open tibial fractures in the paediatric population: a systematic review of the literature. Br Med Bull. 2009;**91**:75–85.

21. **Blasier R, Barnes C.** Age as a prognostic factor in open tibial fractures in children. Clin Orthop. 1996;**331**:261–4.

22. **Robertson P, Karol LA, Rab GT.** Open fractures of the tibia and femur in children. J Pediatr Orthop. 1996;16(5):621–6.

23. **Baldwin KD, Babatunde OM, Russell Huffman G, Hosalkar HS.** Open fractures of the tibia in the pediatric population: a systematic review. J Child Orthop. 2009;3(3):199–208.

24. **Buckley SL, Smith GR, Sponseller PD, Thompson JD, Robertson WW, Jr, Griffin PP.** Severe (type III) open fractures of the tibia in children. J Pediatr Orthop. 1996;16(5):627–34.

Chapter 15

Open Fragility Fractures

Summary

The management of open fragility fractures should follow the established principles as for any open fracture of the lower limb with the following additional considerations:

1. From admission, elderly patients should have a comprehensive orthogeriatric assessment promptly, with ongoing geriatric input throughout their hospital stay, coordinated with related services (e.g. falls prevention, rehabilitation, bone health, mental health, primary care, and social services).
2. Consider the use of regional anaesthetic techniques.
3. Consider the use of angle-stable fixation devices to enhance skeletal fixation in osteoporotic bone.
4. In patients who are frail or whose soft tissues place them at unacceptably high risk of flap failure, or those for whom a lengthy soft tissue reconstruction procedure may be unsafe, alternative surgical strategies should be considered.

Introduction

Open fragility fractures of the lower limb represent an expanding subgroup in whom surgical reconstruction is complicated by poor-quality bone and soft tissues, and whose complex healthcare needs are exacerbated by frailty and the presence of multiple co-morbidities. These challenges are likely to increase as the Office for National Statistics predicts that the number of people aged 75 and over in the UK will rise from 5.2 million in 2014 to 9.9 million in 2039 (1).

The majority of open fragility fractures of the lower limb occur in the tibia and ankle of older women as a result of a fall from standing (2). Despite the low-energy mechanism, there is a high incidence of Gustilo–Anderson III (predominantly IIIA) injuries (3). This reflects the frailty of this patient group and the combined effects that osteoporosis and skin ageing have upon the quality of the bone and integrity of the surrounding soft tissue envelope. Reconstruction is complicated by higher rates of mal-union, non-union, necessity for amputation, and mortality as compared with younger patients with similar injuries (4). These patients frequently have complex ongoing healthcare needs requiring additional support, which influence safe delivery of the established 'best practice' surgical interventions.

Social and healthcare needs

Patients with an open fragility fracture should receive prompt comprehensive orthogeriatric assessment to optimise their peri-operative condition. This input should continue throughout the period of hospitalisation and be coordinated with related services—identifying and planning for ongoing health, social, and rehabilitation needs (e.g. falls prevention, bone health, mental health, primary care, and social services).

Surgery

The management goals of open fragility fractures are the same as for any other open lower limb fracture, delivered by a combined orthoplastic team in a specialist centre with the aim of achieving a stable soft tissue envelope at the time of definitive fracture fixation and within 72 hours of injury. However, this subgroup of patients presents specific challenges that may require some adaptation of established treatment principles. These include the use of regional anaesthetic techniques and alternative modes of peri-operative pain relief to reduce the need for opiate analgesia. The challenges of fracture fixation in osteoporotic bone will be familiar to orthopaedic surgeons; stable fixation through use of locking plates or other similar angle-stable devices may provide more secure fixation than standard techniques. The soft tissue excision should follow the same principles as for any open fracture, but surgeons should appreciate that although the skin wound may be large, open fragility fractures are usually low-energy injuries without severe underlying muscle contusion or periosteal stripping. Large wound extensions may not always be required. Alternatives to complex surgical reconstruction of the open fracture should be considered in light of treating frail patients and those with unacceptably high risks of flap failure (e.g. patients with advanced peripheral vascular and coronary artery disease). For example, acute shortening of the tibia through bone resection may allow primary wound closure in those with transverse wounds that would otherwise require a local or free flap. In some exceptional circumstances, small wounds on the lateral side of the ankle may achieve secondary healing in patients for whom the general condition precludes a more complex procedure. If a local flap is required, this may be raised during the first excision of the wound so that it is 'pre-conditioned' and safer to rotate into the defect at the time of definitive wound cover.

Fine wire circular external fixators have a role in complex fracture patterns or those with significant bone loss. For example, most major trauma centres in the UK will treat between 10 and 30 type C pilon (complete articular) fractures per year (5). These injuries have significant soft tissue disruption compounded if the injury is open. Internal fixation carries a high risk of wound complications and management of such open fractures with fine wire circular fixators minimises the additional iatrogenic trauma to the soft tissues. Whilst the use of such external devices necessitates additional care regimes (e.g. pin site care and frame adjustments) and regular outpatient follow-up to pre-empt problems that may follow the physical incumbrance imposed on mobility, the avoidance of potential deep sepsis from wound complications may avert non-union and amputation. The decision to use such devices for open fragility fractures will need an assessment of benefit and risk as well as consideration of the wider implications of care with the fixator *in situ* and the availability of support services to facilitate this.

The Lower Extremity Assessment Project (LEAP) study (6) showed equivalent functional outcomes for amputation and limb salvage through reconstruction in the most severe tibial fractures at 2 years post-injury but with higher risks of complications, additional surgery, and rehospitalisation in the reconstruction group (6). However, lower limb amputation in the elderly changes the level of mobility drastically as the energy consumption of using a prosthesis, even if at the below-knee level, frequently negates the ability to be independently mobile. Nevertheless, early amputation should be considered where reconstructive options are limited and repeated surgical interventions are unwise in the face of frailty and extensive co-morbidity. The decision to perform an amputation should be with a multidisciplinary team involving orthopaedic and plastic surgical teams, rehabilitation specialists, prosthetists, the patient, their family, and their carers.

Conclusion

The number of open fragility fractures presenting to orthoplastic centres is likely to increase. There will be greater demand on resources to manage this group of patients who have complex health, rehabilitation, and social care needs. Extrapolation of the standards used for adults to the fragility fracture group is appropriate at the current time, with the caveats highlighted earlier. Efforts to carry out high-quality research specifically addressing trauma in the elderly are required to better understand the needs and expectations of this important and growing group of patients.

References

1. **Office for National Statistics.** National population projections. 2015 October. https://www.ons.gov.uk/peoplepopulationandcommunity/populationandmigration/ populationprojections

2. **Court-Brown CM, Biant LC, Clement ND, Bugler KE, Duckworth AD, McQueen MM.** Open fractures in the elderly. The importance of skin ageing. Injury. 2014;**46**(2):189–94.

3. **Court-Brown CMC, Bugler KEK, Clement NDN, Duckworth ADA, McQueen MMM.** The epidemiology of open fractures in adults. A 15-year review. Injury. 2012;**31**(6):891–7.

4. **Clement ND, Beauchamp NJF, Duckworth AD, McQueen MM, Court-Brown CM.** The outcome of tibial diaphyseal fractures in the elderly. Bone Joint J. 2013;**95**-B(9):1255–62.

5. **Sharma H.** Incidence of type c pilon fractures. Unpublished survey data, Hull Royal Infirmary, UK. 2016.

6. **Bosse MJ, MacKenzie EJ, Kellam JF, Burgess AR, Webb LX, Swiontkowski MF, et al.** An analysis of outcomes of reconstruction or amputation after leg-threatening injuries. N Engl J Med. 2002;**347**(24):1924–31.

Chapter 16

Outcome Measures

Summary

1. Core outcomes for patients with open fractures of the lower limb include:
   - quality-of-life
   - return to life roles
   - walking, gait and mobility
   - pain and discomfort.
2. Following a consensus process with patients, healthcare professionals and research methodologists the EuroQol-Five Dimensions-5L and the Lower Extremity Functional Scale are recommend to be used in future studies as a minimum.
3. UK funding bodies expect patient-reported outcome measures to be reported in studies.

What is an outcome measure and an outcome measurement instrument?

Outcome measures are a core component of clinical audit or research and need to encompass information relevant to patients and healthcare professionals. They may measure specific clinical events (e.g. absence or presence of infection) or they may capture a broader domain (e.g. quality of life) to demonstrate effects of an intervention on wider aspects of health (1).

An outcome measure refers to *what* is measured. It is also referred to as a construct, domain, or concept. In a clinical trial it refers to what is being measured on participants to examine the effect of the intervention (2). An outcome measurement instrument (OMI) refers to *how* the outcome is measured. It is a tool to measure the quality or quantity of an outcome (2) (e.g. the Oxford Hip Score). For example, when conducting a trial, the investigators may want to collect information on the quality of life of participants, and thus the outcome measure would be health-related quality-of-life, and this could be collected using an OMI such as the EuroQol-Five Dimensions (EQ-5D-5L), Short Form 36 (SF-36), or Sickness Impact Profile (SIP).

Selection of outcome measures that record the impact of an intervention on appropriate domains of health accurately is difficult. The World Health Organization's International Classification of Functioning, Disability and Health model (ICF) identifies multiple interrelated domains of disability affecting a patient's recovery. In the context of a severe lower limb injury these can be divided into impairments of body functions and structure, together with activity limitations and restrictions to participation that are influenced by the environment and personal factors (3). A common approach to assessing the multi-dimensional aspects of recovery in patients with open fractures of the lower limb is to use multiple outcome measures, aiming to capture different domains of health (4). Consequently, a battery of OMIs are often combined, including both general quality-of-life questionnaires and disease- or limb-specific instruments (5).

Increasingly, outcome measures should be patient-derived in an endeavour to focus on the relevant domains that enable better patient-centred care. The Core Outcomes in Clinical Effectiveness Trials (COMET) initiative promotes efforts to involve stakeholders, including patients, to reach a consensus on the most important outcomes to collect as a minimum in a specified disease entity. This is called a core outcome set (COS), which identifies what outcomes to measure. A Core Outcome Measurement Instrument Set (COMIS) identifies how to measure the COS, i.e. which OMIs to use. By establishing a consensus over what the most important outcomes are and how to measure them, consistency of outcome reporting across trials and clinical audit will be improved (1). In addition, future studies are more likely to measure appropriate outcomes, maximise the potential to contribute to systematic review and meta-analysis, and reduce selective outcome reporting in the future (1).

Different types of outcome measures

Outcome measures can be divided into different types:

1. objective clinical measures
2. patient-reported outcome measures (PROMs)
   a. general health and quality of life
   b. disease/region-specific
3. physical performance measures.

Examples of objective clinical measures

Assessment of severity of femoral and tibial shaft fractures:

1. fracture displacement
2. fracture comminution
3. soft tissue injury
4. energy of injury
5. mangled extremity scores.

Assessment of adverse events—bone and soft tissue healing complications. Commonly used outcome measures in this population have consisted of:

1. time to fracture union
2. malunion
3. infection
4. flap failure
5. secondary amputation.

Past studies have focused on objective clinical measures, but it is increasingly expected that current and future studies will be powered on outcome measures that are proven to be meaningful to patients, e.g. PROMs.

Examples of patient-reported outcome measures

PROMs are questionnaires that elicit responses to measure either patients' perceptions of their general health or function in relation to specific diseases or conditions (6). Responses to questions are scored to provide a quantitative measure of an assumed underlying domain of health, known as the latent trait, which can be used as the estimated instantaneous status of that trait in that patient.

When investigating a specific condition, such as open lower limb fractures, disease- or region-specific PROMs provide a greater clinical focus than generic health measurement instruments as they are tailored to the symptoms and disability of the condition of interest (7). When selecting PROMs, it is essential to ensure they possess a degree of validity. Important components of validity to consider include (8):

◆ Content validity, whether the instrument measures all important domains.
◆ Construct validity, whether the instrument measures what it intends to measure.
◆ Reliability, the extent to which measurements of individuals are similar when obtained in different conditions.

General health outcome measurement instruments

EuroQol-Five Dimensions questionnaire

EQ-5D-5L is a validated, generalisable, and standardised instrument for measuring generic health status (9). It comprises a five-level scale (no problems, slight problems, moderate problems, severe problems, and unable to perform task or extreme pain/anxiety) measuring across five domains related to daily activities: (i) mobility, (ii) self-care, (iii) usual activities, (iv) pain and discomfort, and (v) anxiety and depression (10). The respondent self-rates their health status by marking on a visual analogue scale (EQ-VAS; 0–100), labelled 'best imaginable health state' (100) and 'worst imaginable health state' (0). The EQ-5D-5L can be used to estimate quality-adjusted life-years (QALYs) as part of a health economic analysis and is used by the National Institute of Clinical Care and Excellence (NICE). It is responsive to change both when self-reported (9) and when proxy-reported for patients with cognitive impairment (11). EQ-5D-5L is one of the most commonly used generic questionnaires to measure health-related quality of life, is short and easy to use (taking about 5 minutes to complete), and is validated for use in a wide range of settings (12).

Medical Outcomes Study Short Form 12-Item

The Short Form-12 (SF-12) was developed as a shorter version of the Short Form-36. It uses the same eight subscales (physical functioning, the physical role, pain, general health, vitality, social function, emotional function, and mental health), which can be clustered into physical and mental component scores (13). It yields two summary scores comprising physical function and mental well-being. It was developed in an effort to reduce respondent burden and has proved to be useful in a variety of settings where a short generic health measure of patient-assessed outcome is required (14). The SF-12 was selected as an outcome measure in the UK Wound Management of Open Lower Limb Fractures (WOLLF) trial (HTA 10/57/20) and was used in combination with survival data to facilitate health economic evaluation (15).

Disabilities Rating Index

The Disabilities Rating Index (DRI) is a self-administered, 12-item questionnaire assessing the patient's rating of their disability through assessment of activity and participation limitations (16). The DRI is quick to complete, taking

<5 minutes. The 12 items are measured using a visual analogue scale (VAS 0–100) with low scores denoting little or no disability. The items are grouped into three distinct sections: basic activities of daily life, daily physical activities, and work-related or more vigorous activities (17). Questionnaire items were chosen to be applicable to disability secondary to pain, impairment of hip or knee function, and to impairment of gross body movements from pain, neurological, and muscle pathologies (16). The DRI was shown to be highly reliable with good validity, discriminating between different diagnostic categories. It met the need for responsiveness with good acceptability, practicality, and a high compliance rate (16). The DRI was selected as the primary outcome measure in the WOLLF study owing to its ability to assess 'gross body movements', making it a good choice for assessing patients presenting with a variety of fracture configurations (15).

Sickness Impact Profile

The SIP is a widely used 136-item patient-oriented general health questionnaire that covers domains of physical functioning, psychosocial health, sleeping, and work; it can be self- or interviewer-administered (18, 19). It assesses cognitive, social, emotional, and physical functioning in the performance of many activities of daily life and takes 20–30 minutes to complete (18). The SIP was developed in the 1970s with the intention of providing patient-oriented outcomes beyond the traditional measures of mortality and morbidity across a range of types of illness, severity, and demographic and cultural subgroups (18). The ability of SIP to measure function broadly and be sensitive to less severe outcomes following lower extremity fractures (19) was why it was selected as an outcome measure in the Lower Extremity Assessment Project (LEAP) (20). However, its length may limit practicality for use in routine practice and decrease compliance rates when used for research in the absence of sufficient patient incentive.

Disease- or region-specific outcome measures

A recent systematic review of outcome measurement tools used for leg, ankle, and foot conditions identified 12 distinct OMIs (21). A selection of relevant region-specific OMIs are described in the chapter. The two most validated OMIs identified were the Foot and Ankle Ability Measure (FAAM) and the Lower Extremity Functional Scale (LEFS), represented in two and six studies, respectively (21). Outcome measures described are scored with respect to reliability, content validity, and construct validity in Table 16.1.

Table 16.1 Evidence for frequently used general lower limb and ankle patient-reported outcome measures.
Based on Martin and Irrgang (2007) (25).

Measure	Focus	Reliability	Content validity	Construct validity	MCID
AAOS-FA	Regional	+	+	+	
FAAM	Regional	+	+	+	+
FAOS	Regional	+	+	+	
LEFS	Regional	+	+	+	+

+ denotes presence of validation studies.

MCID, minimal clinically important difference; AAOS-FA, American Academy of Orthopaedic Surgeons lower limb outcomes assessment instruments Foot and Ankle module; FAAM, Foot and Ankle Ability Measure; FAOS, Foot and Ankle Outcome Score; LEFS, Lower Extremity Functional Scale.

Foot and Ankle Ability Measure

The FAAM was designed as a region-specific OMI to evaluate changes in the self-reported physical function for patients with musculoskeletal disorders of leg, ankle, and foot (22). It contains two subscales, a 21-item assessment for activities of daily living (ADL), and an 8-item sports subscale compiled with the intention of providing information across a spectrum of ability. The items are scored using a Likert scale, where higher scores represent better function (22). The FAAM was validated on 1027 patients receiving treatment for leg, ankle, and foot musculoskeletal disorders referred for physiotherapy (22).

Lower Extremity Functional Scale

The LEFS is a broad region-specific OMI suitable for patients with musculoskeletal disorders of the hip, knee, leg, ankle, or foot (23). The LEFS contains 20 items specifically assessing International Classification of Functioning, Disability, and Health model domains of activity and participation. It too uses Likert scales, where a higher score represents better ability (23). The LEFS was originally validated on 107 subjects presenting predominately with knee disorders ($n = 71$) but also included other lower limb impairments, including in the leg ($n = 8$) and thigh ($n = 1$) (23).

American Academy of Orthopaedic Surgeons lower limb outcomes assessment instruments Foot and Ankle module

The American Academy of Orthopaedic Surgeons (AAOS) developed OMIs designed for patients of all ages with musculoskeletal conditions affecting all body regions (24); for example, the AAOS lower limb outcomes Foot and Ankle module (AAOS-FA) is their region-specific OMI for patients with a foot- and ankle-related diagnosis (25). It consists of a lower limb core scale, a global foot and ankle scale, and a shoe comfort scale. The lower limb core scale contains nine items that assess symptoms and functional status (25).

Foot and Ankle Outcome Score

The Foot and Ankle Outcome Score (FAOS) is a region-specific OMI designed to evaluate symptoms and functional limitations in patients with foot and ankle disorders (26) and is adapted from the Knee Injury and Osteoarthritis Outcome Score (27). The FAOS consists of five subscales: pain (nine items), ADL (17 items), sports and recreational activities (five items), foot- and ankle-related quality of life (four items), and other symptoms (seven items). Each subscale is scored separately using a Likert scale where a higher score represents a better function (25, 26).

Physical performance measures

Physical performance measures (PPMs) are defined as clinician-observed measures of physical function that assess a task (28). PPMs of mobility can quantify the ability of an individual with an open lower limb fracture to perform certain tasks that require movement. PPMs focus on the assessment of the ICF domain classed as 'activities' and relate to 'the ability to move around' (29) and 'the ability to perform daily activities' (30) rather than direct tests of body structure, function, or impairment (28). PPMs are often assessed directly by an observer while the activity is being performed by timing, counting, or distance measurement (28). One such method of assessment is the Enneking Score.

Enneking Score

The Enneking Score is a physician-administered OMI that includes functional assessment measures as well as donor site morbidity. It was originally designed to assess pain, function, walking distance, use of aids, gait, and emotional acceptance following musculoskeletal tumour excision and reconstruction (31). It has also been used to assess limb function following reconstruction after severe open tibial fractures (Grade IIIB) (32) and severe open ankle fractures (33). The scoring system contains components for assessment of the lower and upper limb for which the clinician assigns a numerical value (0–5) for each of the six assessment categories based on their clinical judgement. A numerical score and percentage rating is produced, with the final score expressed as a percentage of the patient's uninjured limb, allowing for control of confounding variables (e.g. co-morbidities) (31, 33).

Quantitative physical performance measures

Perhaps the most fundamental goal of functional recovery from an open lower limb fracture is pain-free walking. This can be assessed easily and directly in a variety of ways including a simple 10-meter timed walk test, self-paced walk test, or 6-minute walk test (28). There are also PPMs of other mobility tasks such as the stair climbing, chair stand, and timed up and go tests (28); however, these activities can be viewed as extensions of walking (34). Typically, simple walking measures focus on gait speed, which has been demonstrated to be a strong indicator of pathology (35, 36). This can be performed on patients with cognitive impairments where PROMs may not be feasible. Despite the practicalities of performing simple timed walk tests in the clinic, these are limited by an inability to discriminate between normal and pathological gait in situations where patients adopt a compensatory gait pattern in order to maintain velocity (37). This inability can be overcome by comprehensive gait analysis using modern measurement apparatus, thus enabling the capture of detailed aspects of movement on walking (34). Following lower limb pathology, highlighted by studies of ankle fractures, the main disturbance of walking gait is asymmetry (38, 39). See Table 16.2 for methods of assessing gait asymmetry.

Table 16.2 Methods for assessing gait asymmetry.

Method	Mechanism
Motion Analysis	Measurement of the magnitude and timing of joint movements using body markers to allow multiple cameras to capture 3D motion in a fixed gait analysis laboratory (e.g. VICON®, Oxford, UK)
Force Plates	Force plates are used to quantify ground reaction forces during weight bearing to provide an indication of the functional demands on the foot. Plantar pressure movement is closely related and can identify regions of high pressure between the ground and foot (34)
Electromyography (EMG)	EMG captures coordination and timing of muscle activity
Energy Expenditure	Energy expenditure can be calculated to examine the efficiency of gait mechanics
Temporo-spatial Footfall Analysis	Combines gait muscle kinetics (effect of muscle forces on joints) and arthrokinematics (movement of joints) to provide a robust measure of gait quality (34, 40). This is commonly measured using a walkway containing electronic pressure sensors to capture the spacing and timing of footfalls (e.g. GAITRite®, CIR Symptoms, Havertown, PA) (34)

Many of the methods for assessing gait symmetry described in Table 16.2 are currently not practical for use in routine clinic follow-up of patients with open lower limb fractures as they require specialist training and facilities. However, measuring gait symmetry in the clinic is an increasingly realistic option by use of temporo-spatial footfall analysis systems, and wearable inertial motion sensors, as these systems are portable and increasingly user friendly.

Outcome measures for resource use

There has been little work to date investigating the economic burden to healthcare providers and patients following open lower limb fracture. The LEAP study was a large multicentre prospective cohort study conducted in the United States reporting outcomes from 601 participants who underwent reconstruction or amputation following severe, lower limb trauma (41). The LEAP study made the first detailed economic evaluation of the associated healthcare treatment cost of sustaining an open lower limb fracture by comparing the lifetime cost of reconstruction vs amputation (42). The main drivers of resource use after injury were identified as direct healthcare costs and projected lifetime costs. Direct healthcare costs included the initial hospitalisation, readmissions, inpatient rehabilitation, outpatient clinic, physical and occupational therapy attendances, and prosthetic devices and related services. Projected lifetime costs included projected healthcare costs and projected prosthetic costs (42).

More recently the WOLLF trial conducted a prospective economic evaluation alongside a UK multicentre randomised controlled trial to estimate the cost-effectiveness of negative pressure wound therapy (NPWT) compared with standard dressing in patients following open lower limb fracture (15). A cost-utility analysis was undertaken and expressed in terms of incremental cost attributable to the NPWT per QALY gained as recommended by NICE. The EQ-5D was used to measure health-related quality of life from which utility was valued using the York A1 model derived from a UK population using a time-trade off technique (43). Using this model, responses to each of the five domains in the EQ-5D can be valued on a health utility-scale from −0.59 to 1, where negative values represent health states considered worse than death, 0 being equivalent to being dead, and 1 being in a state of perfect health. The SF-12 was also collected within WOLLF and responses were converted into a form from which QALYs could be calculated.

When measuring and valuing health effects, health effects should be expressed in QALYs. The EQ-5D-3L is the preferred measure of health-related quality of life in adults for NICE (44).

Outcome measurement instruments developed for open lower limb fractures

While generic outcome measures are proven to be valid across multiple disease states and different populations (45–47), their use in measuring outcomes during recovery from injury is disputed (48). It has been recognised that many disease- or region-specific outcome measures used currently in trauma failed to involve patients at the item-generation stage of development (47). It is notable that the tools used focus on the physical aspects of recovery, overlooking the psychosocial impact of an open fracture, such as dealing with scarring and changes in appearance.

This deficit is addressed through the development of a novel patient-centred recovery score for lower limb trauma by a research group based in Swansea, UK. A qualitative approach has been used with the aim to assess how patients perceived their recovery following open tibial fractures (47). Topics of pain and mobility were shown to be central to descriptions of recovery by all patients interviewed. Domains of health additionally identified as important in the patient experience of recovery were sleep, flexibility, temperature (in relation to its effect on symptoms), fear, appearance, employment and finance, recovery, goal setting, adaption, and impact on others. This work has resulted in the creation of the Wales Lower Limb Recovery Scale (WaLLTR), which has undergone validation on patients with open lower limb fractures (49). The WaLLTR scale consists of a Likert and non-Likert section. The Likert section has 10 items covering 8 domains:

1. Self-efficacy
2. Pain
3. Body image
4. Activity participation
5. Fear
6. Social impact
7. Financial considerations
8. Perception of recovery.

Core Outcomes for Open Lower Limb Fracture Study (CO-OLLF)

In March 2019 following COMET guidance, a COS was developed for patients recovering from open lower limb fractures to identify what outcomes to measure. A consensus was reached for four core outcomes:

1. Quality of life
2. Return to life roles (e.g. employment, military duty, caring)
3. Walking, gait, and mobility
4. Pain or discomfort.

Further work identified how these outcomes should be measured in an additional consensus meeting in February 2020 attended by patients, clinicians, and expert methodologists. The OMIs that reached consensus to be included in the COMIS to measure core outcomes were the EQ-5D-5L and the LEFS to measure 'quality of life' and 'walking, gait, and mobility', respectively. Consensus was not achieved to identify an OMI for the core outcomes 'return to life roles' and 'pain or discomfort'. The WaLLTR Scale was considered the best OMI to measure 'return to life roles' but failed to reach a consensus for inclusion in the COMIS. It was recommended that the WaLLTR scale be revised to specifically address measuring 'return to life roles'. OMIs discussed for pain were considered inadequate due to being too non-specific for patients with open fractures, and in particular not addressing the chronic pain element that many patients describe during recovery. Although no OMI was selected for 'return to life roles' or 'pain and discomfort' the EQ-5D-5L does have face validity to measure all four core outcomes.

Conclusion

There is significant variation in outcome measures used in studies to date investigating outcome following treatment of open fractures of the lower limb. The CO-OLLF study addresses this by establishing a COMIS recommending the EQ-5D-5L and the LEFS to be collected as a minimum in all future studies on patients recovering from open lower limb fractures. This will reduce data heterogeneity in future studies and improve research quality.

References

1. Williamson PR, Altman DG, Blazeby JM, Clarke M, Devane D, Gargon E, et al. Developing core outcome sets for clinical trials: issues to consider. Trials. 2012;13(1):132.
2. Prinsen CAC, Vohra S, Rose MR, Boers M, Tugwell P, Clarke M, et al. How to select outcome measurement instruments for outcomes included in a 'Core Outcome Set'—a practical guideline. Trials. 2016;17(1):86. http://www.comet-initiative.org
3. World Health Organization. International Classification of Functioning, Disability and Health (ICF). Geneva: World Health Organization; 2001.
4. Cook C, Queen RM, Slaven EJ, DeOrio JK, Easley ME, Nunley JA. Dimensionality of measures for severe unilateral ankle arthritis. PM&R.; 2010; 2(11):987–94.

5. **Pynsent P, Fairbank J, Carr A.** Outcome Measures in Orthopaedics and Orthopaedic Trauma. Second ed. Boca Raton, FL: CRC Press; 2004.

6. **Dawson J, Doll H, Fitzpatrick R, Jenkinson C, Carr AJ.** The routine use of patient reported outcome measures in healthcare settings. BMJ. 2010;**340**:c186–6.

7. **Black N.** Patient reported outcome measures could help transform healthcare. BMJ. 2013;**346**:f167–7.

8. **McDowell I.** Measuring health: a guide to rating scales and questionnaires. Third ed. New York, NY: Oxford University Press; 2006.

9. **Parsons N, Griffin XL, Achten J, Costa ML.** Outcome assessment after hip fracture: is EQ-5D the answer? Bone Joint Res. 2014;**3**(3):69–75.

10. **Dolan P.** Modeling valuations for EuroQol health states. Med Care. 1997;**35**(11):1095.

11. **Bryan S, Hardyman W, Bentham P, Buckley A, Laight A.** Proxy completion of EQ-5D in patients with dementia. Qual Life Res. 2005;**14**(1):107–18.

12. **Gusi N, Olivares PR, Rajendram R.** The EQ-5D health-related quality of life questionnaire. In: **V Preedy, R Watson** (eds) Handbook of Disease Burdens and Quality of Life Measures. New York, NY: Springer New York; 2010. pp. 87–99.

13. **Ware JE, Sherbourne CD.** The MOS 36-item short-form health survey (SF-36). I. Conceptual framework and item selection. Med Care. 1992;**30**(6):473–83.

14. **Jenkinson C, Layte R.** Development and testing of the UK SF-12 (short form health survey). J Health Services Res Policy. 1997;**2**(1):14–18.

15. **Achten J, Parsons NR, Bruce J, Petrou S, Tutton E, Willett K,** et al. Protocol for a randomised controlled trial of standard wound management versus negative pressure wound therapy in the treatment of adult patients with an open fracture of the lower limb: UK Wound management of Open Lower Limb Fractures (UK WOLFF). BMJ Open. 2015;**5**(9):e009087.

16. **Salén BA, Spangfort EV, Nygren AL, Nordemar R.** The Disability Rating Index: an instrument for the assessment of disability in clinical settings. J Clin Epidemiol. 1994;**47**(12):1423–35.

17. **Parsons H, Bruce J, Achten J, Costa ML, Parsons NR.** Measurement properties of the Disability Rating Index in patients undergoing hip replacement. J Rheumatol. 2015;**54**(1):64–71.

18. **Bergner M, Bobbitt RA, Carter WB, Gilson BS.** The Sickness Impact Profile: development and final revision of a health status measure. Med Care. 1981;**19**(8):787–805.

19. **Jurkovich G, Mock C, MacKenzie E, Burgess A, Cushing B, deLateur B,** et al. The Sickness Impact Profile as a tool to evaluate functional outcome in trauma patients. J Trauma. 1995;**39**(4):625–31.

20. **Webb LX, Bosse MJ, Castillo RC, MacKenzie EJ, LEAP Study Group.** Analysis of surgeon-controlled variables in the treatment of limb-threatening type-III open tibial diaphyseal fractures. J Bone Joint Surg Am. 2007;**89**(5):923–8.

21. **Shultz S, Olszewski A, Ramsey O, Schmitz M, Wyatt V, Cook C.** A systematic review of outcome tools used to measure lower leg conditions. Int J Sports Phys Ther. 2013;**8**(6):838–48.

22. **Martin RL, Irrgang JJ, Burdett RG, Conti SF, Van Swearingen JM.** Evidence of validity for the Foot and Ankle Ability Measure (FAAM). Foot Ankle Int. 2005;**26**(11):968–83.

23. **Binkley JM, Stratford PW, Lott SA, Riddle DL, Network TNAORR.** The Lower Extremity Functional Scale (LEFS): scale development, measurement properties, and clinical application. Physical Ther. 1999;**79**(4):371–83.

24. **Johanson NA, Liang MH, Daltroy L, Rudicel S, Richmond J.** American Academy of Orthopaedic Surgeons lower limb outcomes assessment instruments. J Bone Joint Surg Am. 2004;**86**(5):902–9.

25. **Martin RL, Irrgang JJ.** A survey of self-reported outcome instruments for the foot and ankle. J Orthop Sports Phys Ther. 2007;**37**(2):72–84.

26. **Roos EM, Brandsson S, Karlsson J.** Validation of the foot and ankle outcome score for ankle ligament reconstruction. Foot Ankle Int. 2001;**22**(10):788–94.

27. **Roos EM, Roos HP, Lohmander LS, Ekdahl C, Beynnon BD.** Knee Injury and Osteoarthritis Outcome Score (KOOS)—development of a self-administered outcome measure. J Orthop Sports Phys Ther. 1998;**28**(2):88–96.

28. **Bennell K, Dobson F, Hinman R.** Measures of physical performance assessments: Self-Paced Walk Test (SPWT), Stair Climb Test (SCT), Six-Minute Walk Test (6MWT), Chair Stand Test (CST), Timed Up & Go (TUG), Sock Test, Lift and Carry Test (LCT), and Car Task. Arthritis Care Res. 2011;**63**(S11):S350–70.

29. **Bellamy N, Kirwan J, Boers M, Brooks P, Strand V.** Recommendations for a core set of outcome measures for future phase III clinical trials in knee, hip, and hand osteoarthritis. Consensus development at OMERACT III. J Rheumatol. 1997;**24**(4):799–802.

32. **Naique SB, Pearse M, Nanchahal J.** Management of severe open tibial fractures: the need for combined orthopaedic and plastic surgical treatment in specialist centres. J Bone Joint Surg Br. 2006;**88**(3):351–7.

33. **Khan U, Smitham P, Pearse M, Nanchahal J.** Management of severe open ankle injuries. Plast Reconstr Surg. 2007;**119**(2):578–89.

34. **Perry J, Burnfield JM.** Gait Analysis: Normal and Pathological Function. Second ed. Thorofare, NJ: SLACK Incorporated; 1992.

35. **Studenski S.** Bradypedia: is gait speed ready for clinical use? J Nutr Health Aging. 2009;**13**(10):878–80.

36. **Fritz S, Lusardi M.** White Paper: 'Walking Speed: the Sixth Vital Sign'. J Geriatr Phys Ther. 2009;**32**(2):2.

37. **Kirtley C.** Clinical Gait Analysis. Edinburgh: Elsevier Churchill Livingstone; 2006.

38. **Becker HP, Rosenbaum D, Kriese T, Gerngro H, Claes L.** Gait asymmetry following successful surgical treatment of ankle fractures in young adults. Clin Orthop Relat Res. 1995;**311**:262.

39. **Wang R, Thur CK, Gutierrez-Farewik EM, Wretenberg P, Broström E.** One year follow-up after operative ankle fractures: a prospective gait analysis study with a multi-segment foot model. Gait & Posture. 2010;**31**(2):234–40.

40. **Neumann DA.** Kinesiology of the Musculoskeletal System. St. Louis, MO: Mosby; 2013.

41. **MacKenzie EJ, Bosse MJ.** Factors influencing outcome following limb-threatening lower limb trauma: lessons learned from the Lower Extremity Assessment Project (LEAP). J Am Acad Orthop Surg. 2006;**14**(10 Spec No.):S205–10.

42. **MacKenzie EJ, Jones AS, Bosse MJ, Castillo RC, Pollak AN, Webb LX,** et al. Health-care costs associated with amputation or reconstruction of a limb-threatening injury. J Bone Joint Surg Am. 2007;**89**(8):1685–92.

43. **Dolan P.** Modeling valuations for EuroQol health states. Medical Care. 1997;**35**(11):1095–108.

44. **National Institute for Health and Care Excellence.** Guide to the Methods of Technology Appraisal 2013. London: NICE; 2013.

45. **Dagum AB, Best AK, Schemitsch EH, Mahoney JL, Mahomed MN, Blight KR.** Salvage after severe lower-extremity trauma: are the outcomes worth the means? Plast Reconstr Surg. 1999;**103**(4):1212–20.

46. **Ware JE, Sherbourne CD.** The MOS 36-item short-form health survey (SF-36). I. Conceptual framework and item selection. Medical Care. 1992;**30**(6):473–83.

47. **Trickett RW, Mudge E, Price P, Pallister I.** A qualitative approach to recovery after open tibial fracture: the road to a novel, patient-derived recovery scale. Injury. 2012;**43**(7):1071–8.

48. **Watson WL, Ozanne-Smith J, Richardson J.** Retrospective baseline measurement of self-reported health status and health-related quality of life versus population norms in the evaluation of post-injury losses. Inj Prev. 2007;**13**(1):45–50.

49. **Trickett RW, Mudge E, Price P, Pallister I.** The development of a novel patient-derived recovery scale for open tibial fractures. Bone Joint J. 2020;**11**(1):17–25.

Chapter 17

Patient Experience of Open Fracture and Practical Psychological Support

Summary

1. Psychological difficulties following open fracture are common and should receive attention alongside the physical effects of injury to help improve long-term functioning.

2. Patients require support from trauma teams to express strong emotions, manage their pain, adjust to their wounds, live with limited mobility, and reimagine their future lives.

3. Drawing on cognitive-behavioural therapy (CBT) and eliciting a patient's thoughts, feelings, behavioural choices, and physiological reactions may help validate patient experience and provide information for mental health referral where indicated.

4. Common post-traumatic symptoms will often alleviate over time, but their elevation can be predictive of later post-traumatic stress disorder. Patients experiencing acute stress will benefit from regular orientation to their surroundings and help to focus on daily life.

5. A patient's distress about change in appearance is linked to their subjective perception rather than objective clinical assessment. Patients may require: support to look at and touch scars and flaps; help with anxiety, which may be indicated by excessive checking or avoidance of their wound; and opportunities to discuss their concerns. Neutral descriptors should be used where possible (e.g. change in appearance rather than deformity).

6. Patients should be referred to a trained mental health clinician for evidence-based treatment where their psychological difficulties are negatively impacting their functioning and recovery.

Introduction

In the immediate aftermath of an open fracture, patients are faced with the psychological effect of trauma, sudden hospitalisation, and ongoing physical impairment. Psychological distress in this context is common and can be lasting. Evidence suggests that approximately a third of severely injured adults screen positive for a likely psychological disorder up to 2 years post-injury (1, 2). This is a new diagnosis for many (1), indicating that the impact of injury has a sustained effect on their lives. Evidence from patient experience combined with existing psychological models may provide guidance for appropriate clinical input. This chapter outlines what we know about patient experience of open fracture of the lower limb, considers practical psychological support drawing on cognitive-behavioural principles, and explores two key patient challenges: changes to appearance and heightened psychological distress.

Patient experience

Patient-based evidence underpins clinical guideline development (3) and provides opportunities for developing shared understanding and decision making (4). Interviews with patients whilst in hospital (5) as part of the UK Wound Management of Open Lower Limb Fractures (WOLLF) trial (6) highlight the significant impact of trauma on patients' lives and emotional well-being. The following provides a summary of their experience:

- Participants were shocked by the strength of their emotions, which they had not experienced before, or they compared to feelings they had when a family member died. It felt like an emotional rollercoaster. At the same time, they were controlling their emotions to help their family and friends cope with the impact of their injury.
- Participants talked extensively about their pain, the different types of pain, and approaches to pain control. Many identified a time when they were in extreme pain.
- Participants were horrified by their wounds, skin, and muscle flaps. They were grateful to staff who supported them and helped them to understand what was happening to their legs. However, they needed to feel ready to see their wound for the first time and time to adjust to their wounds, often before showing them to family members.
- Being physically constrained by their injuries was a real struggle for patients; they monitored their bodies and were grateful for a degree of control over their ability to move about but were frustrated by inactivity.

◆ Being able to imagine how their life might continue at home was a challenge for participants. They felt there was a point where they became ready to think about it and visually imagine it. However, they remained anxious about what it would be like and sad about the things they would not be able to do.

In summary, in the early phase of recovery patients with open fracture of the lower limb require support to enable them to: (i) express strong emotions, (ii) manage their pain, (iii) adjust to having wounds, (iv) live with limited mobility, and (v) reimagine their future life.

Later on in recovery, there is some evidence that patients have changed lives and struggle to return to normal or adapt to being disabled. For example, the impact of not being able to bear weight was noted by patients with fractures around the ankle in interviews ($n = 36$) up to 10 weeks post-injury, where they expressed frustration and felt depressed due to inactivity and being confined to a small geographical space (7). In addition, major trauma patients ($n = 15$) at 3–6 months, including those with lower limb injury, identified how they were determined to get better, frustrated by setbacks, wanted to do the right thing but ultimately felt they needed to redefine who they were in order to incorporate their injury into their life (8). Interviews with participants with open lower limb fractures ($n = 9$) up to 2.8 years post-injury suggested they were still struggling, with some not returning to normal (9). In this study, participants identified ongoing pain and stiffness, reduced mobility, fear of falling, concerns about their appearance, and changed finances as affecting their lives. The vulnerability expressed by patients with open fractures of the lower limb suggests that a continued focus on emotional well-being, pain, wound management, mobility, and hopes for the future are important to support patients' recovery from traumatic injury.

Practical psychological support

Emotional support offered to patients who experience closeness to death or loss of limb is embedded in daily hospital activities (10) and is a central part of interventions to reduce distress. Timely assessment of how patients are feeling, their social support, and current coping strategies provides a basis for identifying the specific interventions required. An evidence-based model for carrying out such an assessment can be drawn from cognitive-behavioural therapy (CBT) (11). As a treatment, CBT is one of a number of appropriate models that may be used and it can aid a trauma team's understanding of a patient's response to their injury. The model highlights the interplay between how an individual thinks, feels, and behaves in relation to their physical experience. It is underpinned by recognition that a person's experience of an event, in this case an open fracture, is influenced by their thoughts about it, and these in turn are affected by pre-existing beliefs, which have been shaped by lived experience (12). It is important for the whole trauma team to understand this interplay between the physical injury and the emotional response. By eliciting what a patient is thinking, the team can develop understanding of their emotional responses, behavioural choices, and physiological reactions. Figure 17.1 highlights how each

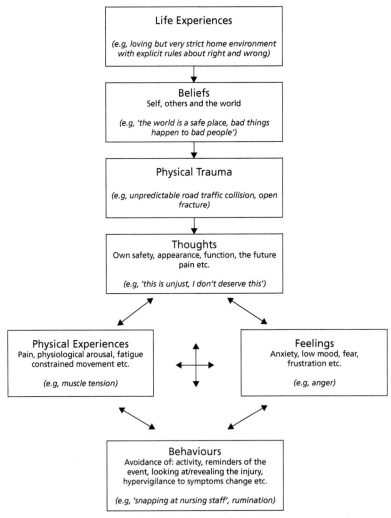

Figure 17.1 To show one way in which the interrelationship between experience, thoughts, beliefs, and behaviour might be approached in recovery from an open fracture of the lower limb.

of these areas influences the others in a reciprocal fashion and has the potential to form a vicious cycle.

A simple way of gathering information within this framework is to ask the patient:

◆ 'What's going through your mind at the moment (thoughts)?'

Followed by questions such as:

◆ 'And when you think this, what feelings come up for you (feelings)?'

◆ 'And what does that lead you to do (behaviours)?'

◆ 'And what sensations do you notice in your body (physical)?'

It is possible to start at any point (thoughts, feelings, behaviours, physical sensations) in this mini-formulation depending on the prominent experience for the patient. For example, 'You're looking worried, can you tell me what thoughts are going through your mind when we talk about your next operation?' The thoughts and feelings shared may echo those identified in patient experience research, and valuable emotional support for the patient at this stage can be to reflect and summarise what they say; for example:

> My understanding from what you have said is that when you hear that another operation may be necessary [trigger], you feel scared [feelings], your body tenses up [physical sensations], you worry that you are going to remain in hospital for a long time and that you may never fully recover [thoughts], and you feel frustrated [feelings] that you aren't making the progress you had anticipated [thoughts]. All this makes it harder for you to try the exercises the physiotherapist has given you and you often decline their sessions [behaviours].

Acknowledging patient experience in this way is a form of psychological support accessible to all clinical staff, and for those patients where significant psychological distress is identified it provides referral information for assessment and intervention by an appropriately trained mental health practitioner.

Key challenges

This way of interacting with patients may be used to explore some of the key challenges faced by those with an open fracture, such as changes to appearance and heightened psychological distress.

Changes to appearance

Open fractures are often associated with large wounds and flaps. An ongoing task for the patient is therefore adjustment to the loss of their previous appearance, development of the confidence to manage any potential social stigma, and engagement in valued living. Injury severity and objective clinical assessment of visible change are not associated with patient-reported levels of appearance distress (13). Instead, the patient's perception of disfigurement noticeability serves as a more accurate predictor (14). Crucially, such perceptions are amenable to psychological input (15). Supporting a patient to look at and (when appropriate) touch their scars and flaps is a valuable step towards encouraging reintegration of their altered body image into their sense of self. It is helpful to talk with patients about their thoughts and images prior to looking at their wounds and to be observant for avoidance or excessive checking, which may maintain anxiety. Sensitive use of ongoing photographs can be a valuable way of shared monitoring of the healing process (16). Patient concerns about how the injury looks should be openly discussed and medical vocabulary carefully chosen to avoid inadvertently alienating them (e.g. correction, deformity). Later in the recovery process, questions about how noticeable the patient believes the injury to be and whether this is a worry to them or leads to avoidance will help to legitimise potential concerns (13).

Heightened psychological distress

There are a number of relevant points to consider in relation to psychological distress in this group of patients. These are:

◆ The association between psychological distress and ongoing disability is strong (17), and indeed the psychological well-being of trauma patients has a greater influence than pain or injury severity on their longer-term functioning post-trauma (18, 19), even after controlling for baseline mental health (20).

◆ It is acknowledged that pain control post-surgery can be difficult to manage (21) and is often underestimated (22). There is evidence that psychological factors (including depression, anxiety, and pain catastrophising) play an important role in patient experience of acute pain and increase risk for the transition from acute to chronic pain (23).

◆ Anxiety and depression may be more common in open than closed fractures (17, 24). Such conditions tend to reduce a person's capacity to actively manage their fracture and this predicts lowered functioning over time (25). Staff can support such concerns through realistic hopefulness, where they focus on what is possible in the short term and help the patient to develop achievable goals (26).

◆ Alongside mood changes, it is important to remember that immediately after a traumatic injury such as an open fracture, patients will often report some post-traumatic symptoms (5). For a minority, these symptoms may elevate over time and this is predictive of subsequent post-traumatic stress disorder (PTSD) and depression (27).

- It should also be acknowledged that those experiencing acute stress will believe themselves to be in continued danger. Orientation to current surroundings will therefore frequently be necessary.

- Within an acute trauma setting, appropriate psychometric screening tools should be readily available, e.g. the Posttraumatic Adjustment Scale (28) and a referral route to psychology and psychiatry established. At subsequent outpatient appointments, a variety of self-report psychometric measures can be used to highlight ongoing psychological difficulty. A high incidence of post-traumatic stress symptoms among patients with severe lower limb trauma has been noted in this context (29).

- Ongoing research continues to highlight different possible early interventions for PTSD (30, 31) and National Institute for Health and Care Excellence (NICE) [NG116] now recommends trauma-focused CBT for adults with acute stress disorder or clinically important PTSD symptoms *within* the first month post-trauma. In addition, the depression and anxiety so often associated with limb fractures may be alleviated using evidence-based therapeutic techniques provided by trained clinicians (32, 33).

Conclusion

To conclude, patient experience research highlights the vulnerability expressed by patients with open fractures of the lower limb and suggests that a continued focus on emotional well-being, pain and wound management, mobility, and hopes for the future may aid a patient's recovery. Trauma teams can support patients by being aware of patient concerns, proactive in creating an environment in which patients can express their emotions, enquiring about their well-being, normalising their experience and being alert to their need for additional support or treatment. Future research on patient experience needs to explore recovery trajectories and investigate which patient-focused interventions that incorporate emotional well-being are most effective, for whom, and under what circumstances.

References

1. Bryant RA, O'Donnell ML, Creamer M, McFarlane AC, Clark CR, Silove D. The psychiatric sequelae of traumatic injury. Am J Psychiatry. 2010;**167**(3):312–20.
2. McCarthy ML, MacKenzie EJ, Edwin D, Bosse MJ, Castillo RC, Starr A, et al. Psychological distress associated with severe lower-limb injury. J Bone Joint Surg Am. 2003;**85**-A(9):1689–97.

3. **Staniszewska S, Boardman F, Gunn L, Roberts J, Clay D, Seers K,** et al. The Warwick Patient Experiences Framework: patient-based evidence in clinical guidelines. Int J Qual Health Care. 2014;**26**(2):151–7.

4. **CG138 NCG.** Patient Experience in Adult NHS Services: Improving the Experience of Care for People Using Adult NHS Services. London: National Clinical Guideline Centre, 2012.

5. **Tutton EA, J. Lamb, SE. Willett, K. Costa, M.** on behalf of the UK WOLLF research collaborators. A qualitative study of the experience of an open fracture of the lower limb in acute care. Bone Joint J. 2018;**100-B**:522–6.

6. **Costa ML, Achten J, Bruce J,** et al. Effect of negative pressure wound therapy vs standard wound management on 12-month disability among adults with severe open fracture of the lower limb: the WOLLF Randomized Clinical Trial. JAMA. 2018;**319**(22):2280–8.

7. **Keene DJ, Mistry D, Nam J, Tutton E, Handley R, Morgan L,** et al. The Ankle Injury Management (AIM) trial: a pragmatic, multicentre, equivalence randomised controlled trial and economic evaluation comparing close contact casting with open surgical reduction and internal fixation in the treatment of unstable ankle fractures in patients aged over 60 years. Health Technol Assess. 2016;**20**(75):1–158.

8. **Claydon JH, Robinson L, Aldridge SE.** Patients' perceptions of repair, rehabilitation and recovery after major orthopaedic trauma: a qualitative study. Physiotherapy. 2017;**103**(3):322–9.

9. **Trickett RW, Mudge E, Price P, Pallister I.** A qualitative approach to recovery after open tibial fracture: the road to a novel, patient-derived recovery scale. Injury. 2012;**43**(7):1071–8.

10. **Tutton E, Seers K, Langstaff D.** Professional nursing culture on a trauma unit: experiences of patients and staff. J Adv Nurs. 2008;**61**(2):145–53.

11. **Greenberger DP, CA.** Mind Over Mood: Change How You Feel By Changing the Way You Think. Second edn. New York, NY: Guildford Press; 2015.

12. **Beck A.** Cognitive Therapy for Depression. New York, NY: Guildford Press; 1979.

13. **Rumsey N, Clarke A, Musa M.** Altered body image: the psychosocial needs of patients. Br J Community Nurs. 2002;**7**(11):563–6.

14. **Lansdown RR, N. Bradbury, E. Carr, T. Partridge, J.** Visibly Different: Coping with Disfigurement. Boca Raton, FL: CRC Press; 1997.

15. **Rumsey N, Harcourt D.** Body image and disfigurement: issues and interventions. Body Image. 2004;**1**(1):83–97.

16. **NG37 NCG.** Fractures (Complex): Assessment and Management. London: NICE; 2016.

17. **Crichlow RJ, Andres PL, Morrison SM, Haley SM, Vrahas MS.** Depression in orthopaedic trauma patients. Prevalence and severity. J Bone Joint Surg Am. 2006;**88**(9):1927–33.

18. **O'Donnell ML, Varker T, Holmes AC, Ellen S, Wade D, Creamer M,** et al. Disability after injury: the cumulative burden of physical and mental health. J Clin Psychiatry. 2013;**74**(2):e137–43.

19. **Starr AJ.** Fracture repair: successful advances, persistent problems, and the psychological burden of trauma. J Bone Joint Surg Am. 2008;**90**(Suppl 1):132–7.

20. Michaels AJ, Michaels CE, Smith JS, Moon CH, Peterson C, Long WB. Outcome from injury: general health, work status, and satisfaction 12 months after trauma. J Trauma. 2000;**48**(5):841–8; discussion 8–50.

21. Eriksson K, Wikstrom L, Fridlund B, Arestedt K, Brostrom A. Patients' experiences and actions when describing pain after surgery—a critical incident technique analysis. Int J Nurs Stud. 2016;**56**:27–36.

22. Seers T, Derry S, Seers K, Moore RA. Professionals underestimate patients' pain: a comprehensive review. Pain. 2018;**159**(5):811–18. DOI: 10.1097/j.pain.0000000000001165

23. Mcgreevy K, Bottros MM, Raja SN. preventing chronic pain following acute pain: risk factors, preventive strategies, and their efficacy. Eur J Pain Suppl. 2011;**5**(2):365–72.

24. Giannoudis PV, Harwood PJ, Kontakis G, Allami M, MacDonald D, Kay SP, et al. Long-term quality of life in trauma patients following the full spectrum of tibial injury (fasciotomy, closed fracture, grade IIIB/IIIC open fracture and amputation). Injury. 2009;**40**(2):213–19.

25. Wegener ST, Castillo RC, Haythornthwaite J, Mackenzie EJ, Bosse MJ, Group LS. Psychological distress mediates the effect of pain on function. Pain. 2011;**152**(6):1349–57.

26. Tutton E, Seers K, Langstaff D. Hope in orthopaedic trauma: a qualitative study. Int J Nurs Stud. 2012;**49**(7):872–9.

27. Mellman TA, David D, Bustamante V, Fins AI, Esposito K. Predictors of post-traumatic stress disorder following severe injury. Depress Anxiety. 2001;**14**(4):226–31.

28. O'Donnell ML, Creamer MC, Parslow R, Elliott P, Holmes AC, Ellen S, et al. A predictive screening index for posttraumatic stress disorder and depression following traumatic injury. J Consult Clin Psychol. 2008;**76**(6):923–32.

29. Bhat W, Marlino S, Teoh V, Khan S, Khan U. Lower limb trauma and posttraumatic stress disorder: a single UK trauma unit's experience. JPRAS. 2013; **67**(4): 555–60

30. Kearns MC, Ressler KJ, Zatzick D, Rothbaum BO. Early interventions for PTSD: a review. Depress Anxiety. 2012;**29**(10):833–42.

31. O'Donnell ML, Lau W, Tipping S, Holmes AC, Ellen S, Judson R, et al. Stepped early psychological intervention for posttraumatic stress disorder, other anxiety disorders, and depression following serious injury. J Trauma Stress. 2012;**25**(2):125–33.

32. CG90 NCG. Depression in Adults: Recognition and Management. London: NICE; 2009.

33. CG113 NCG. Generalised Anxiety Disorder and Panic Disorder in Adults: Management Guideline. London: NICE; 2011.

Chapter 18

Rehabilitation After Severe Open Tibial Fractures

Summary

1. Rehabilitation in major trauma centres (MTCs) should be delivered by a multidisciplinary team (MDT) led by a consultant in rehabilitation medicine.

2. Patients with an isolated open tibial fracture should be assessed by a member of the MDT and provided with a rehabilitation prescription (RP) within two calendar days of admission.

3. Patients requiring inpatient rehabilitation (usually for injuries other than their open tibial fracture) should be assessed by the inpatient unit within 10 days.

4. The weight-bearing status of the limb and permissible range of movement of joints (with respect to both bony stability and soft tissue reconstruction) must be recorded in the clinical notes and RP immediately after definitive surgical treatment. Unrestricted rehabilitation should be the goal of surgery and achieved as early as possible.

5. The patient's recovery after severe open tibial fracture should be assessed 12 months after injury using the EuroQol-Five Dimensions (EQ-5D) tool.

6. A member of the rehabilitation MDT should have the ability to screen patients for post-traumatic stress disorder (PTSD); ideally the team should include a clinical psychologist.

7. Referral to a specialist pain medicine service should be considered if pain symptoms are becoming chronic, are not related to a treatable cause, and are persisting despite treatment by the surgical team and GP.

8. A patient undergoing delayed amputation should have a peri-operative pain control plan in place prior to surgery.

9. A patient undergoing delayed amputation should be assessed by a prosthetist or a consultant in rehabilitation medicine prior to surgery.

10. Surgeons should consider referring patients with poorly functioning but reconstructed lower limbs for dynamic orthotics.

11. Patients with a high trans-femoral amputation who do not tolerate standard prosthetic sockets could be considered for osseointegration.

Introduction

Sustaining a severe open tibial fracture is a life-changing injury regardless of whether the eventual clinical outcome is amputation or limb reconstruction (1). Surgical treatment is only the first stage of the patient's recovery. For the patient to achieve their maximum potential for physical, social, and psychological function, greatest participation in society, and quality of living, they require a combination of training and therapy collectively referred to as rehabilitation (2).

After initial surgical treatment there are a finite number of possible clinical outcomes ranging from the surgical objective of infection-free bony union and healed wounds and a useful limb, to primary amputation in an unreconstructable limb. Between these two outcomes is a spectrum of limbs requiring ongoing treatment for infection and/or problems with healing of bones and soft tissues. Those that suffer with persistent complications/consequences of injury may end up with a delayed amputation. The goals for rehabilitation, however, must remain the same, namely to maximise the return of limb functionality and to help integrate the patient back into society by facilitating optimal quality of life. Aside from the limb injury, patients may well have other injuries, e.g. traumatic brain injuries or pre-existing medical co-morbidities, and therefore each patient's rehabilitation needs will vary considerably.

There is a lack of prospective interventional trial data on rehabilitation following open tibial fracture. However there are sufficient observational studies together with trials from related fields, e.g. neuro-rehabilitation, to allow clinical standards and recommendations to be developed. The standards presented in this chapter are consistent with those proposed by the National Institute for Health and Care Excellence (NICE) (3), the British Society of Rehabilitation Medicine (BSRM) (2), the NHS Clinical Advisory Group Trauma (Trauma-CAG) (4), and those adopted by the National Clinical Audit of Specialist Rehabilitation following Major Injury (NCASARI) (5).

Rehabilitation services

The Trauma-CAG identified rehabilitation services as a central component of the formation of the Major Trauma Network (4). Rehabilitation in major trauma centres (MTCs) should be delivered by a multidisciplinary team (MDT) led by a consultant in rehabilitation medicine (2–4).

The BSRM standards for major trauma recommend that all trauma casualties with an Injury Severity Score (ISS) ≥9 (i.e. an isolated open tibia fracture) be assessed by a member of the MDT and provided with an initial rehabilitation prescription (RP) within two calendar days of admission (2), which can be finalised after definitive skeletal fixation and soft tissue reconstruction. The minimum surgical input to the RP should include clear direction regarding the weight-bearing status of the limb and the permissible range of movement of the adjacent joints. This should be agreed jointly by orthopaedic and plastic surgeons, and clearly documented at each stage of surgical treatment. To facilitate rehabilitation, the default position after definitive surgery should be no restrictions on either joint movement or weight-bearing, i.e. 'weight-bearing as tolerated'. The reason for and time limits of any restrictions should be clearly documented.

It is anticipated that most patients with isolated open tibial fractures will require a basic RP, which will be delivered on an outpatient basis. However, those with more complex treatment needs, concurrent injuries, or significant medical co-morbidities will require a specialist RP and may well need inpatient rehabilitation (5). Patients requiring inpatient rehabilitation should be assessed by the inpatient unit within 10 days.

Measuring outcomes

This is covered in greater detail in Chapter 16. Units treating open tibial fractures should measure their results alongside submission of data to the Trauma Audit Research Network (TARN) (6). Measuring outcomes offers a surrogate of the performance of a unit and drives quality improvement efforts.

Outcome measures should be valid, i.e. actually measure the outcome of interest, and standardised to not only allow a unit to determine trends in their own performance over time, but also permit comparisons between units (7).

Infection

Infection following open tibial fracture is associated with amputation and fixation failure (8), and the rate of infection is cited as a surrogate marker of unit performance (9). For this measure to be meaningful a clear definition of infection must be employed and the time period over which infection surveillance occurs specified.

There remains no accepted definition of 'infection', with studies employing various definitions, including positive microbiological specimens (10), clinical diagnosis (9), a requirement for surgical treatment (8), or the use of diagnostic criteria. The most commonly used diagnostic criteria is the US Centers for Disease Control (CDC) surgical site infection tool (11), though the recently proposed fracture-specific tool from Metsemakers *et al.* (12) should be considered for future use.

Amputation rate

The rate of amputation following severe open tibial fracture, often regarded as synonymous with 'failed reconstruction', has also been cited as an outcome measure (9). However, this is problematic as it assumes reconstruction is always the superior outcome, a position not supported by multiple studies that have found either similar or superior patient-reported outcomes following amputation (1, 13–15). The use of amputation rates as an outcome measure in isolation should be avoided and surgeons should continue to base complicated discussions with patients regarding amputation and reconstruction on the likely best outcome for the individual patient.

Patient-reported outcome measures

It is now accepted practice to measure the success of medical treatment at least in part on the patient's perception of the results of the intervention. Following open tibial fracture, the main choice is between using an anatomic-specific measure, i.e. looking at knee or ankle function, or a general health-related quality-of-life (HRQOL) measure (15). There is currently no specific outcome measure for measuring recovery after tibia fracture.

The main HRQOL measures used following orthopaedic trauma are the Short Form-36 (SF-36) (15), the Sickness Impact Profile (SIP) (16), and the EQ-5D (17). The main disadvantage of these tools is that concurrent injuries, e.g. traumatic brain injury, will be reflected in the overall outcome measure, and not just the effect of the lower limb injuries. An advantage over anatomic-specific patient-reported outcome measures (PROMs) is that general HRQOL measures are applicable both to patients who retain their limbs and those who undergo amputation.

SF-36 has been the most widely used measure in studies of orthopaedic trauma, but its use normally incurs a cost, whereas SIP and EQ-5D are available on an open-use basis for non-commercial purposes.

EQ-5D is the HRQOL outcome measure used by NHS England in the PROMs programme (18), and is therefore recommended as the generic PROM for assessing recovery following open tibial fracture. It is known that PROMs will change for years after injury (1), and so an arbitrary 12-month point is recommended for recording EQ-5D scores.

Psychological impact

The physical effects of a severe extremity injury are obvious, however the damage to mental health can also be profound. This is examined in greater detail in Chapter 17. The events surrounding a life-changing injury such as an open tibial fracture are frequently so outside normal experience as to result in psychological injury.

The Lower Extremity Assessment Project (LEAP) group detailed the prolonged psychological impact of a lower limb-threatening injury persisting 7 years after injury (1, 19). The psychological effect for children with severe lower limb injuries was documented by Levy et al., who interviewed 40 paediatric patients with open tibial fractures. A quarter of these patients continued to suffer from flashbacks and nightmares involving the events of the accident.

A study by Bhat et al. (20) looked specifically at post-traumatic stress disorder (PTSD) following open tibial fracture. This study used the Post-Traumatic Stress Disorder Checklist Scale (PCL), a validated scoring system based on the Diagnostic and Statistical Manual IV definition of PTSD. The study showed that in a cohort of 60 patients who had sustained an open tibial fracture and who had undergone successful limb reconstruction, 30% of patients suffered from PTSD. The other significant finding in this study was that patients younger than 50 years of age were at greater risk of PTSD. The authors speculated that the events producing the higher energies required to fracture younger bone might be more traumatic than those resulting in lower-energy injuries in older patients.

Whilst the majority of patients do not suffer long-term psychological consequences following their injury, there should be provision within rehabilitation MDTs for screening for PTSD using simple tools like the PCL. Ideally a clinical psychologist should be a (usually part-time) member of the rehabilitation MDT (21). If this is not possible, then the rehabilitation MDT's occupational therapist should be trained to screen for PTSD and a referral pathway to local clinical psychology services established.

Chronic pain

Limb-threatening injuries and the surgical treatments required to manage them are potent pain stimuli. The management of acute pain is a core skill of a surgeon treating these injuries, but it is recognised that for some patients painful symptoms can become more complex and persist beyond the point where the surgical goals of fracture union and wound closure have been achieved.

Identifying chronic pain is challenging. The Royal College of Anaesthetists (RCA) defines complex pain as 'Any pain associated with, or with the potential to cause, significant disability and/or distress' (22). The point at which acute pain evolves into more complex chronic pain is poorly understood (23) and there is no defined time point at which pain symptoms can be regarded as becoming 'chronic'.

The persistence of painful symptoms after treatment for an open tibial fracture occurs after both amputation (24) and reconstruction (25), and is closely associated with, and regarded as a driver of, poor functional recovery (26). The LEAP study reported approximately 20% patients with severe chronic pain 7 years after open tibia fracture (27). In a US study of opioid prescription it was found that 20% of patients who received surgery for a lower limb injury were still using controlled opiate analgesia 3 months after injury (28). In the European Chronic Pain Survey 18% of patients in the UK with chronic pain cited a traumatic injury as the cause of their symptoms (29).

The causes of pain symptoms are as heterogeneous as the limb injuries themselves. Pain following reconstruction is associated with fracture non-union (30), prominent metal work (31), post-traumatic arthritis (32), intra-medullary nail entry point (33), free tissue transfer, nerve damage (34), or often a combination of these factors. Conversely, pain following amputation is usually associated with nerve transection, neuroma (35), or prosthetic fitting issues, such as bony prominence, heterotopic ossification, or soft tissue mobility (36).

Surgeons managing patients with limb-threatening injuries should recognise that the effective control of acute pain is probably the most effective way to prevent the development of chronic and complex pain (23).

Surgeons treating patients with ongoing pain symptoms after severe lower limb fractures should first identify and treat any potentially amenable anatomic cause of pain symptoms (22). Second, they should recognise the development of chronic and complex pain symptoms and identify the need for onward referral to specialist pain services.

The RCA Core Standards on Pain Medicine Service (22) recommend that referral of patients to specialist pain services following severe lower limb injury should be considered in the following circumstances:

1. Patients with persistent or recurrent pain not adequately managed by surgical team in conjunction with the patient's GP.
3. Patients whose pain is causing significant distress or functional impairment.
4. Patients with analgesic misuse problems or who are taking recreational drugs/alcohol for pain relief.
5. Patients with pain-related psychological and psychosocial problems (e.g. pain-related fear, anxiety, reactive depression, functional impairment) that complicate their pain symptoms or rehabilitation.

In the specific case of limb amputation performed following unsuccessful reconstruction, patients should have preoperative anaesthetic assessment and a pain control plan written for the peri-operative period. Consideration should be given to the use of peri-neural catheterisation (37) or epidural infiltration (38) of analgesic and anaesthetic agents.

Prosthesis and orthotics

The use of a prosthetic to replace function or an orthotic to augment it is commonly required after severe lower limb trauma.

In the case of amputation, the prosthetist's role in the patient's rehabilitation is fundamental. When limb amputation is not being performed as an urgent procedure, the patient should be assessed by the rehabilitation consultant or prosthetist prior to surgery (39). This allows the patient to be informed about the likely timing and sequential manner of prosthetic fitting, along with the expected rehabilitation process.

Whilst the role of prosthetics following amputation is obvious, there is increasing evidence that orthotics may significantly improve function after limb reconstruction and retention. It is recognised that in patients with limb-threatening injuries, particularly those involving the foot and ankle, outcomes after limb reconstruction can be inferior to amputation (14).

The development of energy-storing and returning orthotics occurred as part of the effort to improve rehabilitation in US service personnel with severely injured but reconstructed limbs (40), and has been shown to significantly improve outcomes after reconstruction (41). Surgeons should consider referring patients with poorly functioning reconstructed lower limbs for dynamic orthotics.

Osseointegration

The transfer of forces between the skeleton and the prosthesis occurs at the interface between the prosthesis socket and the residual limb. This can frequently be a reason for pain and difficulty with prosthetic use as a result of poor soft tissues, heterotopic ossification, and bony prominence (42). Osseointegration allows for the direct transfer of forces from the skeleton to the prosthesis, bypassing the soft tissue envelope of the residual limb.

In 1990 Brånemark et al. implanted the first osseointegrated mount for a prosthetic coupling in a trans-femoral amputee (43). Since then techniques and implants have improved and osseointegration has developed from an experimental technique to a valid, albeit specialist, treatment modality (44).

It is recommended that patients with a high trans-femoral amputation who do not tolerate standard prosthetic sockets be referred to a specialist centre with experience in osseointegration.

References

1. MacKenzie EJ, Bosse MJ, Pollak AN, Webb LX, Swiontkowski MF, Kellam JF, et al. Long-term persistence of disability following severe lower-limb trauma. Results of a seven-year follow-up. J Bone Joint Surg Am. 2005;87(8):1801–9.
2. British Society of Rehabilitation Medicine. Specialist Rehabilitation in the Trauma Pathway: BSRM Core Standards. London: Royal College of Physicians; 2013.
3. NICE. Trauma—Quality Standards (QS166). London: NICE; 2018.
4. Report NCAG. Regional Networks for Major Trauma. London: NHS; 2010.
5. National Clinical Audit of Specialist Rehabilitation following Major Injury. Specialist rehabilitation for patients with complex needs following major trauma. London: National Clinical Audit of Specialist Rehabilitation following Major Injury; 2016.
6. TARN. Trauma Audit and Research Network Manchester 2018. : https://www.tarn.ac.uk/Content.aspx?ca=4
7. Bryant D, Fernandes N. Measuring patient outcomes: a primer. Injury. 2011;42(3):232–5.
8. Penn-Barwell JG, Bennett PM, Fries CA, Kendrew JM, Midwinter MJ, Rickard RF. Severe open tibial fractures in combat trauma: management and preliminary outcomes. Bone Joint J. 2013;95-B(1):101–5.
9. Wordsworth M, Lawton G, Nathwani D, Pearse M, Naique S, Dodds A, et al. Improving the care of patients with severe open fractures of the tibia: the effect of the introduction of Major Trauma Networks and national guidelines. Bone Joint J. 2016;98-B(3):420–4.
10. Johnson EN, Burns TC, Hayda RA, Hospenthal DR, Murray CK. Infectious complications of open type III tibial fractures among combat casualties. Clin Infect Dis. 2007;45(4):409–15.
11. Mangram AJ, Horan TC, Pearson ML, Silver LC, Jarvis WR. Guideline for Prevention of Surgical Site Infection, 1999. Centers for Disease Control and Prevention (CDC) Hospital Infection Control Practices Advisory Committee. Am J Infect Control. 1999;27(2):97–132; quiz 3–4; discussion 96.
12. Metsemakers WJ, Morgenstern M, McNally MA, Moriarty TF, McFadyen I, Scarborough M, et al. Fracture-related infection: a consensus on definition from an international expert group. Injury. 2018;49(3):505–10.
13. Doukas WC, Hayda RA, Frisch HM, Andersen RC, Mazurek MT, Ficke JR, et al. The Military Extremity Trauma Amputation/Limb Salvage (METALS) study: outcomes of amputation versus limb salvage following major lower-extremity trauma. J Bone Joint Surg Am. 2013;95(2):138–45.
14. Bennett PM, Stevenson T, Sargeant ID, Mountain A, Penn-Barwell JG. Outcomes following limb salvage after combat hindfoot injury are inferior to delayed amputation at five years. Bone Joint Res. 2018;7(2):131–8.

15. **Busse JW, Jacobs CL, Swiontkowski MF, Bosse MJ, Bhandari M.** Complex limb salvage or early amputation for severe lower-limb injury: a meta-analysis of observational studies. J Orthop Trauma. 2007;**21**(1):70–6.

16. **Bergner M, Bobbitt RA, Kressel S, Pollard WE, Gilson BS, Morris JR.** The sickness impact profile: conceptual formulation and methodology for the development of a health status measure. Int J Health Serv. 1976;**6**(3):393–415.

17. **EuroQol.** EuroQol—a new facility for the measurement of health-related quality of life. Health Policy. 1990;**16**(3):199–208.

18. **NHS England.** National PROMS Programme Guidance. Leeds: NHS; 2017.

19. **McCarthy ML, MacKenzie EJ, Edwin D, Bosse MJ, Castillo RC, Starr A, et al.** Psychological distress associated with severe lower-limb injury. J Bone Joint Surg Am. 2003;**85-A**(9):1689–97.

20. **Bhat W, Marlino S, Teoh V, Khan S, Khan U.** Lower limb trauma and posttraumatic stress disorder: a single UK trauma unit's experience. J Plast Reconstr Aesthet Surg. 2014;**67**(4):555–60.

21. **Centre for Work Force Intelligence.** NHS Clinical Advisory Group on Major Trauma Workforce. London: NHS; 2011.

22. **Faculty of Pain Medicine.** Core Standards for Pain Management Services in the UK. London: Royal College of Anaesthetists; 2015.

23. **Lavand'homme P.** The progression from acute to chronic pain. Curr Opin Anaesthesiol. 2011;**24**(5):545–50.

24. **Penn-Barwell JG.** Outcomes in lower limb amputation following trauma: a systematic review and meta-analysis. Injury. 2011;**42**(12):1474–9.

25. **Harries L, Emam A, Khan U.** Pain after ortho-plastic reconstruction of lower limb injuries: a snapshot study. Injury. 2018;**49**(2):414–19.

26. **Vallier HA, Cureton BA, Patterson BM.** Factors influencing functional outcomes after distal tibia shaft fractures. J Orthop Trauma. 2012;**26**(3):178–83.

27. **Castillo RC, MacKenzie EJ, Wegener ST, Bosse MJ, Group LS.** Prevalence of chronic pain seven years following limb threatening lower extremity trauma. Pain. 2006;**124**(3):321–9.

28. **Holman JE, Stoddard GJ, Higgins TF.** Rates of prescription opiate use before and after injury in patients with orthopaedic trauma and the risk factors for prolonged opiate use. J Bone Joint Surg Am. 2013;**95**(12):1075–80.

29. **Breivik H, Collett B, Ventafridda V, Cohen R, Gallacher D.** Survey of chronic pain in Europe: prevalence, impact on daily life, and treatment. Eur J Pain. 2006;**10**(4): 287–333.

30. **Antonova E, Le TK, Burge R, Mershon J.** Tibia shaft fractures: costly burden of nonunions. BMC Musculoskelet Disord. 2013;**14**:42.

31. **Brown OL, Dirschl DR, Obremskey WT.** Incidence of hardware-related pain and its effect on functional outcomes after open reduction and internal fixation of ankle fractures. J Orthop Trauma. 2001;**15**(4):271–4.

32. **Buckwalter JA, Brown TD.** Joint injury, repair, and remodeling: roles in post-traumatic osteoarthritis. Clin Orthop Relat Res. 2004(423):7–16.

33. **Toivanen JA, Vaisto O, Kannus P, Latvala K, Honkonen SE, Jarvinen MJ.** Anterior knee pain after intramedullary nailing of fractures of the tibial shaft. A prospective,

randomized study comparing two different nail-insertion techniques. J Bone Joint Surg Am. 2002;**84**-A(4):580–5.

34. **Harris AM, Althausen PL, Kellam JF, Bosse MJ, Castillo R.** Complications following limb-threatening lower extremity trauma. J Orthop Trauma. 2009;**23**(1):1–6.

35. **Ehde DM, Czerniecki JM, Smith DG, Campbell KM, Edwards WT, Jensen MP, et al.** Chronic phantom sensations, phantom pain, residual limb pain, and other regional pain after lower limb amputation. Arch Phys Med Rehabil. 2000;**81**(8):1039–44.

36. **Dillingham TR, Pezzin LE, MacKenzie EJ, Burgess AR.** Use and satisfaction with prosthetic devices among persons with trauma-related amputations: a long-term outcome study. Am J Phys Med Rehabil. 2001;**80**(8):563–71.

37. **Borghi B, D'Addabbo M, White PF, Gallerani P, Toccaceli L, Raffaeli W, et al.** The use of prolonged peripheral neural blockade after lower extremity amputation: the effect on symptoms associated with phantom limb syndrome. Anesth Analg. 2010;**111**(5):1308–15.

38. **Lambert A, Dashfield A, Cosgrove C, Wilkins D, Walker A, Ashley S.** Randomized prospective study comparing preoperative epidural and intraoperative perineural analgesia for the prevention of postoperative stump and phantom limb pain following major amputation. Reg Anesth Pain Med. 2001;**26**(4):316–21.

39. **British Society of Rehabilitation Medicine.** Amputee and Prosthetic Rehabilitation—Standards and Guidelines. London: British Society of Rehabilitation Medicine; 2003.

40. **Patzkowski JC, Blanck RV, Owens JG, Wilken JM, Blair JA, Hsu JR.** Can an ankle-foot orthosis change hearts and minds? J Surg Orthop Adv. 2011;**20**(1):8–18.

41. **Highsmith MJ, Nelson LM, Carbone NT, Klenow TD, Kahle JT, Hill OT, et al.** Outcomes associated with the intrepid dynamic exoskeletal orthosis (IDEO): a systematic review of the literature. Mil Med. 2016;**181**(S4):69–76.

42. **Webster JB, Hakimi KN, Williams RM, Turner AP, Norvell DC, Czerniecki JM.** Prosthetic fitting, use, and satisfaction following lower-limb amputation: a prospective study. J Rehabil Res Dev. 2012;**49**(10):1493–504.

43. **Brånemark R, Brånemark PI, Rydevik B, Myers RR.** Osseointegration in skeletal reconstruction and rehabilitation: a review. J Rehabil Res Dev. 2001;**38**(2):175–81.

44. **Al Muderis M, Khemka A, Lord SJ, Van de Meent H, Frolke JP.** Safety of osseointegrated implants for transfemoral amputees: a two-center prospective cohort study. J Bone Joint Surg Am. 2016;**98**(11):900–9.

Chapter 19

Special Circumstances: Blast, Ballistics, and Mass Casualties

Summary

1. Blast and ballistic mechanisms of injury result in wounds that have different characteristics from those usually seen by orthoplastic teams.

2. Wound severity is proportional to the energy transferred and degree of contamination.

3. The amount of tissue damage may be significantly greater than the size of the obvious wound and is likely to evolve over time.

4. There is a greater likelihood of a systemic response than from other injury mechanisms and particular emphasis must be placed on general supportive care.

5. Perform initial wound surgery as early as feasible in the damage control process.

6. Repeated wound excision is often required in contrast to other mechanisms of injury.

7. Do not primarily close blast or complex ballistic wounds.

8. The decision to use complex reconstruction early should be made more cautiously than with other mechanisms.

9. In mass casualty incidents there might be difficulty in timely access to orthoplastic services and standard treatment pathways may need to be modified to provide a more population-based approach.

10. There are evidence preservation and forensic implications when dealing with these wounds.

Introduction

Blast wounds are caused by variable combinations of the products of explosions (1):

♦ A shock wave.

♦ An expanding energetic mass of hot gases.

♦ Objects propelled by the explosion.

♦ Further damage from effects such as collapsing structures and fires.

Ballistic wounding refers to injuries caused by objects, often termed projectiles, flying through the air and then interacting with tissues. This includes bullets (2) and fragments energised by blast (1).

Since 2001 the UK military have gained significant and effective expertise in managing ballistic and blast injuries (3, 4). This hard-won knowledge has been shared with civilian practitioners and utilised in managing victims of terrorist attacks (5). Future attacks involving a range of wounding mechanisms, including blast and ballistic weapons, are inevitable (6). Therefore, it is vital that civilian practitioners understand how to manage the casualties produced by these types of mechanisms.

Survivable blast and ballistic injuries disproportionately involve the limbs, frequently resulting in complex open fractures (3, 7). This chapter will highlight the management of these injuries, including features associated with mass casualty incidents. The fundamental principles and methods of treatment are essentially the same as injuries encountered in usual practice but they need to be applied in a manner that is mindful of some unique features.

Features of ballistic and blast wounds that must be considered in any treatment plan are:

♦ The overall severity of the wound is related to the energy transferred and the amount of contamination.

♦ High-energy transfer wounds can cause massive amounts of tissue destruction, resulting in complex wounds that are typically heavily contaminated.

♦ The majority of blast wounds will include penetration by fragments.

♦ Blast effects may have systemic physiological consequences.

♦ Blast may drive contamination along tissue planes away from the wound.

♦ Blast effects on tissues may cause progressive necrosis and a 'wound in evolution'.

♦ Bullet wounds have little or no blast component.

- High-energy transfer bullet wounds will have a wider zone of injury than is immediately apparent.
- Low-energy transfer bullet wounds may have little damage beyond the obvious tract.
- If the bullet is still present in the limb it means all of its energy will have been transferred, although it may also represent a bullet that lost most of its energy before impact.
- If the bullet itself has fragmented, or it has fractured bone, it is more likely that the energy transferred to the limb will have been high (8).
- All projectile penetration will have led to a degree of contamination, which may include biological material.

Knowledge of the method of wounding does not directly inform what injuries may have been sustained. The critical factor in determining the extent of damage is the amount of energy transferred. A bullet may pass through thigh muscle transferring little energy leaving only a simple tract, but if it strikes bone all its energy will be dissipated, resulting in a devastating injury (8).

Initial assessment and care

The standard approach to general trauma care should be followed but with an appreciation that patients exposed to blast and ballistic mechanisms are more likely to have sustained widespread injuries.

- Primary survey with heightened awareness of the need for haemorrhage control. This should include a whole body computed tomography (CT) scan, except for the most minor of isolated distal injuries (9).
- A secondary survey with special attention to identify subtle wounds. Even in the absence of clinical signs of a fracture, if a CT scan has not been performed, orthogonal plain radiographs are mandatory; projectiles can penetrate bone without causing discontinuity and bullet fragmentation is a significant finding. Using radio-opaque markers over the surface wounds is useful to predict likely bullet tracts and to plan surgery (10).
- A tertiary survey once a patient is fully aware with a review of all imaging and reports as a definitive check to exclude missed injuries.

Anticipate that the patient will exhibit a generalised systemic reaction to blast injuries with a similar degree of physiological derangement as seen with large burns. It is highly likely that patients from a blast incident will require critical care.

Surgical management

General principles

The key question in the surgical management of projectile wounds is whether this is a low-energy transfer wound, which could be described as benign, or has there been high-energy transfer, i.e. a complex wound?

Features suggestive of high-energy transfer are (8, 11):

- A large (>3 cm diameter) ragged skin defect or surface wound.
- Obvious significant tissue disruption or destruction.
- A large (>3 cm diameter) cavity in muscle.
- Evidence of bone strike, including multi-fragmentary fractures.
- Fragmentation or retention of a projectile.
- Compartment syndrome.

A wound is complex irrespective of energy transfer if the following are seen:

- It has been directly caused by blast.
- Injuries to nerves, vessels, and tendons that require repair.
- Fractures.
- Significant contamination.
- Systemic effects of blast.

Not all markers of complexity are absolute; a degree of surgical judgement is required and this is best informed by experience. The safest option is to have a low threshold for assuming any projectile wound is complex.

All wounds suspected of being complex should undergo surgical assessment under appropriate anaesthesia in an operating theatre. Successful reconstruction will depend on getting the wound assessment correct and this should be thought of as providing a 'wound diagnosis'. This requires a more extensive approach than might be implied by simply using the term wound excision or debridement. The section on 'Initial Wound Surgery' describes this procedure.

In the critically ill trauma patient, priority should be given to applying damage control principles to halt blood loss, minimise contamination, and improve the physiology. *Initial Wound Surgery* may not be the first surgery in this sequence of interventions. However, due to the level of contamination complex ballistic and blast wounds should be addressed as soon as possible.

Imminently life- or limb-threatening injuries

Victims of blast and ballistic injuries have a greater risk of life- or limb-threatening vascular injury compared with more usual mechanisms. When associated with an open fracture the suggested order of surgical intervention is:

1. Rapid temporary control of haemorrhage. In the limb this is most often achieved with a tourniquet. If open surgical access is required to stem haemorrhage both proximal and distal vascular control are needed; often best achieved away from the wound.

2. Fasciotomies. Other required procedures all take time and compartment pressure will be rising. Releasing the compartments can be achieved very rapidly and is best done before blood flow is restored.

3. Formal surgical exposure of the injured vessel segment and temporary vascular shunting if indicated.

4. Full wound assessment, decision making, and wound excision.

5. Initial skeletal stabilisation, usually by external fixation.

6. Definitive vascular repair.

If during this sequence physiological control of the patient is not achieved the procedure should be truncated using damage control surgery principles.

Initial wound surgery

For ease of description the various components of acute surgical management are discussed in a sequence. In reality they are often performed simultaneously.

Most victims of blast are covered with dirt; the social wash should cover the entire body. This also gives an opportunity to check for other wounds.

Wound extension and release

Excise the skin edge of the defect minimally but adequately. Injured tissue will extend beyond the apparent area of damage and this will swell. To permit the swelling to occur without raising the tissue pressures, the skin and fascial envelope need to be incised to extend the wound beyond the obvious zone of injury. This is the original meaning of the term debridement—to unbridle, or release, the wound. In the leg there should be an extremely low threshold for formally releasing all four compartments as described in Chapter 11. Wound extension incisions should be made along the lines of election for fasciotomies. Where wounds are not close to these lines or there are several wounds, use judgement to plan the skin and fascial extensions such that the desired release is complete without sacrificing reconstructive options. Raise the skin and fascial extensions as a single unit in the sub-fascial plane to ensure they constitute a robust flap rather than degloved skin.

Wound exploration and assessment

Wound extension facilitates full wound exploration, which is essential for complete assessment of the wound. All damaged structures need to be identified and the exposure should be wide enough to permit this. Avoid dividing non-injured muscle horizontally to open up a tract; gain access to the deeper parts of the wound by splitting muscle longitudinally.

Wound excision

With an evolving wound, excision of non-viable tissue and contamination is likely to be multi-staged. The aim is to get macroscopic clearance at the first procedure but pragmatically a point is reached where chasing every last small piece prolongs the operative time for minimal benefit. Dubiously viable tissue may improve and, ideally, excision should be limited to definitely non-viable tissue. Detailed evaluation of tissue can take time; in the physiologically unstable patient or in a mass casualty event the threshold may shift to a more rapid and necessarily radical excision.

Bullets and small metallic fragments can be left in limb wounds without detriment. Attempts to retrieve them may cause additional injury. Exceptions to this are where they are intra-articular or impinge on movement and these should be removed. Environmental contamination, particularly non-metallic, tends to cause abscess formation if left. If minor, this does not always progress to invasive infection. The contamination driven up tissue planes by blast tends to impregnate adventitial layers and is not easily wiped off or irrigated out. This normally requires sharp excision of connective tissue.

There are no peculiarities of blast or ballistic injury that alter the decision making on bone viability but extensive periosteal stripping in high-energy-transfer wounds and deep impregnation of contamination should be anticipated. In common with all wounds, copious irrigation after wound excision is essential.

Initial skeletal stabilisation

Stabilising the fracture conveys stability to the soft tissue envelope and reduces infection. This is usually achieved using external fixation. It is preferable to have pins entering the bone through intact skin but this may not be possible with some defects. If wounds are extensive, temporary stabilisation with an internal plate can be performed, anticipating that this will be revised at definitive surgery.

Limb salvage decisions

Definitive decisions about amputation should not be made at initial wound surgery. Definitely non-viable tissue is excised, and if this results in ablation of the limb, then that should be viewed as a wound excision and not an amputation (12). No attempt should be made to influence decision making on skin excision based on trying to plan for specific amputation levels, i.e. all viable skin should be retained until the definitive closure. Similarly, the presence of a fracture should not influence amputation level; fractures proximal to the amputation level can be fixed in the presence of adequate soft tissue cover.

No immediate closure or repairs

No matter how clean or small the wound appears after appropriate initial wound surgery, for complex ballistic and all blast wounds, immediate wound closure is contraindicated. Vascular repairs require cover with viable tissue and this should be achieved by formally mobilising tissue rather than trying to achieve coverage with tension. It is essential that such tissue is only loosely placed to cover the repair and it must not impede free drainage or restrict wound swelling.

Repairs of functional structures such as nerves and tendons, definitive bony fixation, and soft tissue reconstruction must all be delayed until the wound has fully evolved to reveal the full extent of non-viability.

Dressings

There is no conclusive evidence to inform decisions on any specific dressing that might be best for ballistic and blast wounds (13). Nearly a decade of collective military experience in using Kerlix AMD™ gauze in a topical negative pressure dressing has shown it to be excellent for managing large complex three-dimensional wounds in long evacuation chains. The main benefits were ease of nursing and patient comfort. The observation of more rapid wound stabilisation has not been subject to trials.

Non-complex wounds

Wounds that have no evidence of features suggesting complexity, particularly small isolated bullet wounds, can be managed in a relatively conservative manner; the laying open of such wounds is not necessary (8, 11). This involves:

+ Minimal, if any, excision of damaged skin edge.
+ Confirmation that, if deep fascia has been breached, the underlying muscle looks healthy. This may require a minimal extension of the fascial defect.
+ Irrigation of the wound augmented by physical agitation using gauze as a mild abrasive along the wound tract, so-called flossing.
+ A simple dressing.
+ Delayed primary closure or healing by secondary intention.

Forensic considerations

A full description of all wounds including exact size and location must be documented. Virtually all ballistic and blast events will be subject to investigation and this information will constitute evidence. Avoid making any comment on opinions as to the causation of wounds and reference to if a wound is an entrance or exit. This may well be interpreted as an expert assessment of direction of fire and can have very significant legal ramifications. Simply describe what is seen. Removed bullets and other fragments should be retained in such a manner as to make them admissible as evidence. It is best to try and avoid using grasping metal instruments directly to extract bullets as this can alter surface markings of forensic importance. It is recommended that hospitals develop a protocol for the management of evidential material.

Microbiological aspects

There is no evidence that blast or ballistic factors directly influence the species types of microbiological contamination, although the likelihood of deeply penetrating contamination is higher. The prophylaxis regime described in Chapter 1 will suffice for isolated limb injuries. For wider injuries, Public Health England (PHE) have published antimicrobial prophylaxis guidelines for bomb blast victims (14). Any subsequent evidence of infection should prompt the collection of deep tissue samples for prolonged culture and histological analysis. The request form should clearly state that the wound is as a result of an explosion and investigation for fungal species requested; most laboratories now have automated systems that will not culture for unusual organisms unless specifically requested.

There is a possibility that projectiles may pass through other victims. Dismembered body parts may become projectiles. This presents a risk of inoculating wounds with biological matter that carries viable viral material. PHE have published specific guidelines for managing this risk (14).

Second look

A return to theatre for another thorough wound exploration should be planned for about 48 hours. It will be unusual to have to extend wounds further but all wound recesses need to be revisited. It should be anticipated that some further excision of non-viable tissue will be required. The presence of necrotic muscle is not necessarily a reflection of poorly judged initial excision; it is part of the process of wound evolution. It is unusual to see evidence of invasive infection at this stage. Even at this early stage, pus like exudate is seen around residual contamination, although this is nearly always sterile. This phenomenon helps identify and remove the contamination.

Approaches to reconstruction

Patients may well require critical care for prolonged periods and physiological fragility has been observed to persist for many months. The impact of repeated surgical and anaesthetic interventions should not be downplayed.

There are no absolute contraindications to specific methods of reconstruction due to the wound being sustained by blast or ballistic mechanisms. The fact the wound may still be evolving and the patient systemically unwell means that decisions on method and timing of reconstruction may have to be made well past the advocated timeframes described elsewhere in this book.

The aim remains to get the wound closed as early as is safe but the chosen method must be compatible with the patient's condition. Rather than continue with dressings until the patient can tolerate complex reconstruction, it may be preferable to use quick and simple techniques early (such as split skin grafting and external fixation) and accept that revision reconstruction is likely several months later.

Once wound progression appears to have stopped it may become apparent that local flaps are a safe simple option if the patient remains too unwell for a free flap. It should be appreciated that, in the case of a systemic response to blast, the whole body is effectively the zone of injury. The concept of reconstructing from outside the zone of injury is therefore relative. An experienced microvascular surgeon should be able to assess the suitability of a vessel for microsurgical anastomosis by direct visualisation under magnification.

Fracture fixation

There is evidence that bone healing is impaired following ballistic and blast injury and the risk of infection is greater (15). These factors need to be considered when making decisions on definitive skeletal fixation. Fixation constructs should be planned with the assumption of delayed union and therefore suitably robust to be load-bearing for a prolonged time. An exception to this is in the case of tibia fractures with large soft tissue loss. In these instances, a thin, unreamed nail can be placed as an 'internal fixator' to rapidly confer some stability, allowing soft tissue reconstruction. This can then be revised to a larger, stiffer-reamed nail once the soft tissue envelope had matured.

Experience from managing combat casualties

During recent conflicts, several hundreds of blast wounded service personnel were treated by a single UK hospital over more than a decade (3, 4). Certain approaches to management emerged through experiential learning and became regular practice based on recurring success. Although not subject to clinical trials and based on a specific cohort, some of the learning points are likely to be applicable when managing such injuries in a civilian situation (16).

- ◆ In patients too unwell for complex reconstruction, injured tissues were encouraged back to anatomical alignment gradually by using a combination of topical negative pressure dressings and elasticated vascular sloops in a 'bootlace' fashion. This was not used as a primary method of achieving wound closure.

♦ New appearance of significant progressive necrosis (as opposed to small marginal areas) raised suspicion of fungal infection. In this case excised tissue was sent for histological examination as well as microbiological culture.

♦ Each anaesthetic has an impact; patients were not taken back to theatre just to see how wounds were progressing. There had to be a reconstructive goal for each theatre trip, even if only to reduce the size of the wound. The interval between theatre trips was often about 5 days, with topical negative pressure dressing remaining undisturbed in the interval.

♦ Topical negative pressure dressings were used as a means of controlling wound exudate and splintage, particularly of skin grafts. There was no intent to try and make non-graftable wounds graftable by producing granulation tissue.

♦ In general, early wound cover was advocated. Rather than waiting for the patient to become sufficiently stable for complex reconstruction, this was often achieved by a combination of staged delayed primary closure, meshed split skin grafting, and by rearrangement of the flaps raised during wound extensions—so-called flaps of opportunity.

♦ Biosynthetic dermal templates (Integra™ or Matriderm™) took extremely well on muscle and resulted in very pliable amputation stumps.

♦ Some early free flaps were used with success. If the patient was still requiring inotropic support, free flaps were not considered.

♦ In patients with amputations and a requirement for free flaps, consideration was given to donor site morbidity. Latissimus dorsi and rectus abdominus flaps in particular compromise core strength impacting on future mobility and rehabilitation.

♦ The principle of achieving prompt rigid fixation to allow early mobilisation is nugatory if the severity of the injuries made it likely that the patient would not be rehabilitating rapidly. In this situation minimalistic bone fixation was achieved in a manner that reduced further insult to the soft tissue envelope through minimal exposure; for example, with a single lag screw and small neutralisation plate.

Mass casualty incidents

NHS England (and similar applies for the health services of the devolved administrations) defines a mass casualty incident for the health services as an incident (or series of incidents) causing casualties on a scale that is beyond the normal resources of the emergency and healthcare services' ability to manage. Unlike major incidents, mass casualty incidents are infrequent; the last one in the UK probably being the multiple London bombings on 7 July 2005 (17).

Normal major incident planning requires trauma-receiving hospitals that are part of a trauma network predicting in advance how many cases they can deal with in a given timeframe such that normal care pathways can be followed. This would imply that the recommendations for managing complex limb injuries described throughout this publication could be adhered to in a major incident. The major incident plan should include a mechanism to distribute cases such that a single hospital is not burdened beyond its declared capacity. Although it would seem sensible to ensure all complex open fractures would only be taken to those hospitals with an orthoplastic service, there is no formal requirement for this to be the case. Under major incident circumstances there should be opportunities for secondary transfers soon enough to allow compliance with these standards.

When the volume of cases overwhelms the major incident plan, a mass casualty situation exists (18). This is likely to occur when numbers are in the hundreds and in this situation an adjustment to normal clinical pathways is required. Major trauma centres may be filled up with multiply injured patients and isolated, albeit complex, limb injuries could be triaged for transfer to trauma units. Because of the scale of the event, secondary transfer of these patients to facilities with orthoplastic services may not be feasible for many days.

Not all mass casualty incidents will involve blast and ballistic mechanisms. Worldwide, sudden onset natural disasters generate the greatest number of casualties but these are unlikely in the UK. Terrorists have used blunt trauma mechanisms to inflict scores of injuries by driving vehicles into crowds. Historical patterns suggest that about 25% of casualties will need immediate life-saving interventions, 25% will need essential interventions that can wait, and 50% will be walking wounded or minor injuries.

The recommendations in this publication are focused on achieving the best possible outcomes for the individual patient. In a mass casualty scenario the emphasis shifts to a more population-based approach. A crude example would be the difference between using an all-day list to perform a complex reconstruction for a single patient or, instead, amputate that limb and do several more simple reconstructions on many patients. Similarly, the conversion of temporary external fixation to a definitive modality may have to be delayed beyond what is normally considered ideal.

Essential surgical procedures take precedent and the completeness of the first surgical intervention may be truncated. In true damage control surgery the amount of intervention is limited by the patient's physiological condition. In a mass casualty incident an additional limit is access to resources, which includes the availability of surgical teams and operating theatres. Even a physiologically stable patient may have their surgery limited and this is more accurately referred to as abbreviated surgery. This means that at the end of the first surgical intervention, initial wound surgery may not have been completed and this must be clearly documented. If possible, at least gross contamination should be removed from wounds. Antibiotics will still need to be administered but this does not replace the need for surgery. All wounds at some point, even if delayed, must undergo initial wound surgery.

A requirement in the early phases of a mass casualty incident, which may extend into many days, is to be as efficient as possible with the available resources. The main surgical contribution to this is to avoid having to unnecessarily repeat work. It is important to not let the heat of the moment force rushed decisions that impact on later workload.

Approaches that help manage resources include:

- Senior and expert decision making is essential. Be very wary of delegating procedures to unsupervised inexperienced surgeons.
- In the presence of large numbers of surgical patients, a slightly more aggressive approach to tissue excision may be required to reduce the risk of subsequent urgent, unplanned take-backs.
- A surgical command team should keep track of all cases requiring ongoing surgery so there is oversight of the workload. Twice daily surgical planning meetings involving representatives of all relevant specialties should allocate appropriate patients to appropriate resources. To assist this, accurate documentation is essential to record what has been done but also why it was done and what has not been done.
- Do not burden the system with unnecessary changes of dressings and wound inspections. Choose a dressing regime that can be left in place for many days. Every trip to theatre must be planned to make progress with the wounds.
- Be responsive to the patient's general condition; unexplained deterioration may indicate wound issues that could require a return to theatre.
- Immediate wound closure is contraindicated (this does not included providing viable cover for certain tissues).
- Do not commence on definitive reconstruction until wound evolution appears to have ceased.
- Do not make decisions on definitive amputation levels too early.

If specific features of wounding patterns are beyond the normal experience of the treating teams, they should not be reticent in seeking assistance from external sources. There is a formal system in place to enable military aid to the civil authorities, which is requested through the incident command chain, but this is unlikely to be able to yield an additional workforce to deliver clinical care. What is more effective is making available niche expertise for advice and guidance. This was successfully demonstrated following the Manchester bombing of June 2017; a team of combined military and civilian experts from Queen Elizabeth Hospital Birmingham, who had extensive experience in managing blast injured military patients, made visits to involved hospitals to discuss patient pathways and clinical dilemmas (5).

References

1. Breeze J, Ramasamy A. Fragmenting munitions. In: J Breeze, JG Penn-Barwell, D Keene, DJ O'Reilly, J Jeyanathan, PF Mahoney (Eds). Ballistic Trauma—A Practical Guide. London: Springer; 2017.
2. Penn-Barwell JG, Helliker AE. Firearms and bullets. In: J Breeze, JG Penn-Barwell, D Keene, DJ O'Reilly, J Jeyanathan, PF Mahoney (Eds). Ballistic Trauma—A Practical Guide. London: Springer; 2017.
3. Chandler H, MacLeod K, Penn-Barwell JG, Severe Lower Extremity Combat Trauma Study G. Extremity injuries sustained by the UK military in the Iraq and Afghanistan conflicts: 2003–2014. Injury. 2017;48(7):1439–43.
4. Maitland L, Lawton G, Baden J, Cubison T, Rickard R, Kay A, et al. The role of military plastic surgeons in the management of modern combat trauma: an analysis of 645 cases. Plast Reconstr Surg. 2016;137(4):717e–24e.
5. Kerslake Panel. The Kerslake Report: an independent review into the preparedness for, and emergency response to, the Manchester Arena attack on 22nd May 2017; 2018.
6. Security Service. Terrorist Methods London 2018. https://www.mi5.gov.uk/terrorist-methods.
7. Norton J, Whittaker G, Kennedy DS, Jenkins JM, Bew D. Shooting up? Analysis of 182 gunshot injuries presenting to a London major trauma centre over a seven-year period. Ann R Coll Surg Engl. 2018;100(6):464–74.
8. Penn-Barwell JG, Sargeant ID, Severe Lower Extremity Combat Trauma Study G. Gunshot injuries in UK military casualties—features associated with wound severity. Injury. 2016;47(5):1067–71.
9. Dick EA, Ballard M, Alwan-Walker H, Kashef E, Batrick N, Hettiaratchy S, et al. Bomb blast imaging: bringing order to chaos. Clin Radiol. 2018;73(6):509–16.
10. Brooks A, Bowley DM, Boffard KD. Bullet markers—a simple technique to assist in the evaluation of penetrating trauma. J R Army Med Corps. 2002;148(3):259–61.
11. Penn-Barwell JG. Ballistic trauma-considerations for the orthoplastic surgical team. Int J Orthoplast Surg. 2018;1(2):47–54.
12. Penn-Barwell JG, Kendrew J, Sargeant ID. Amputation. In: J Breeze, JG Penn-Barwell, D Keene, DJ O'Reilly, J Jeyanathan, PF Mahoney (Eds). Ballistic Trauma—A Practical Guide. London: Springer; 2017.

13. **Fries CA, Ayalew Y, Penn-Barwell JG, Porter K, Jeffery SL, Midwinter MJ.** Prospective randomised controlled trial of nanocrystalline silver dressing versus plain gauze as the initial post-debridement management of military wounds on wound microbiology and healing. Injury. 2014;45(7):1111–16.

14. **Public Health England.** Antimicrobial Prophylaxis Guidance for Bomb Blast Victims. London: Public Health England; 2017.

15. **Penn-Barwell JG, Bennett PM, Fries CA, Kendrew JM, Midwinter MJ, Rickard RF.** Severe open tibial fractures in combat trauma: management and preliminary outcomes. Bone Joint J. 2013;95-B(1):101–5.

16. **Evriviades D, Jeffery S, Cubison T, Lawton G, Gill M, Mortiboy D.** Shaping the military wound: issues surrounding the reconstruction of injured servicemen at the Royal Centre for Defence Medicine. Philos Trans R Soc Lond B Biol Sci. 2011;366(1562):219–30.

17. **Aylwin CJ, Konig TC, Brennan NW, Shirley PJ, Davies G, Walsh MS,** et al. Reduction in critical mortality in urban mass casualty incidents: analysis of triage, surge, and resource use after the London bombings on July 7, 2005. Lancet. 2006;368(9554):2219–25.

18. **NHS England.** Concept of Operations for managing Mass Casualties. London: NHS England; 2017.

Chapter 20

Setting Up an Effective Orthoplastic Service

Summary

1. The National Institute for Health and Care Excellence (NICE) defined an orthoplastic centre as: 'A hospital with a dedicated, combined service for orthopaedic and plastic surgery in which consultants from both specialties work simultaneously to treat open fractures as part of regular, scheduled, combined orthopaedic and plastic surgery operating lists. Consultants are supported by combined review clinics and specialist nursing teams.'

The BAPRAS/BOA group recommend that for clarity this narrative description of an orthoplastic service by NICE is broken into its component parts as follows:

   - A combined service of orthopaedic and plastic surgery consultants.
   - Sufficient combined operating lists with consultants from both specialties to meet the standards for timely management of open fractures.
   - Scheduled, combined review clinics for severe open fractures.
   - Specialist nursing teams able to care for both fractures and flaps.

In addition, an effective orthoplastic service will also:

   - Submit data on each patient to the Trauma Audit Research Network (TARN).
   - Hold regular clinical audit meetings with both orthopaedic and plastic surgeons present.

2. The most cost-effective treatment strategy, if it can be achieved, is wound excision, definitive fixation, and definitive soft tissue reconstruction as a combined surgical procedure within 24 hours of injury.

3. There are several models in evolution throughout the UK, but the development of the orthoplastic unit is least challenging in hospitals with co-location of trauma orthopaedic surgery and plastic surgery departments.

4. It is vital to establish an adequately resourced service by engaging with specialised (NHS England or equivalent) and non-specialised commissioners (clinical commissioning groups) to support the service and ensure that the treating centres are appropriately reimbursed for delivering optimal care.

Introduction

Open fractures can be both limb-threatening injuries and devastating. The true incidence is difficult to ascertain, although it is estimated that open fractures comprise 3.2% of all fractures (1), with up to 21% of tibial fractures being open. Open fractures are more common in older people, with $296.6/10^6$/year in those aged under 65 years compared with $323.3/10^6$/year in those aged over 65 years, and $446.7/10^6$/year in over 80-year-olds (2, 3). Fracture distribution curves demonstrate a bimodal form with similar incidence in the young male population, 15–19 years of age, and females >90 years of age. Only 22.3% of all open fractures are a result of high-energy injuries (3) and most often affect young adults at their most productive time of life. Although the total number of patients with open fractures is relatively small compared with the total number of fractures treated each year, open fractures cause significant morbidity and represent an enormous burden on healthcare resources. Healthcare providers, managers, and clinicians have a duty to improve outcomes and use resources efficiently.

In 2016, the National Institute for Health and Care Excellence (NICE) published guidance for trauma (4, 5). The Quality Standard from NICE includes a statement on the management of complex open limb trauma, recommending an 'orthoplastic approach' to treatment (6).

NICE defined an orthoplastic centre as:

> A hospital with a dedicated, combined service for orthopaedic and plastic surgery in which consultants from both specialties work simultaneously to treat open fractures as part of regular, scheduled, combined orthopaedic and plastic surgery operating lists. Consultants are supported by combined review clinics and specialist nursing teams (4).

The British Association of Plastic, Reconstructive and Aesthetic Surgeons/ British Orthopaedic Association (BAPRAS/BOA) group recommend that for clarity this narrative description of an orthoplastic service by NICE is defined in its component parts as follows:

- A combined service of orthopaedic and plastic surgery consultants.
- Sufficient combined operating lists with consultants from both specialties to meet the standards for timely management of open fractures.
- Scheduled, combined review clinics for severe open fractures.
- Specialist nursing teams able to care for both fractures and flaps.

In addition, an effective orthoplastic service will also:

- Submit data on each patient to TARN.
- Hold regular clinical audit meetings with both orthopaedic and plastic surgeons present.

For some hospitals managing patients with open fractures, such a strict definition of an orthoplastic service would signal a major change from their current infrastructure. This may cause concern as wholesale service changes would need to be implemented to achieve this new standard, at a cost that few hospitals could afford. Furthermore, there is no prescriptive template for such a service due to variations across the NHS in the UK, as well as a differing approach to trauma delivery between the home nations. However, the coordinated treatment plan defined by the combined approach results in expeditious care of the patient. Hospitals that have established orthoplastic services have demonstrated reductions in deep infection rates that offer cost savings that would be attractive to underfunded healthcare systems (7).

There is evidence that outcomes of these patients are greatly improved with combined orthoplastic management at a designated centre, within defined time frames (5) compared with sequential treatment by separate specialties often within different hospitals. As well as reduced infection rates, improved outcomes include lower rates for non-union and amputation (7, 8), fewer unnecessary trips to theatre both for planning definitive treatment and revision surgery (9–11), reduction in time to soft tissue coverage (8, 10, 12, 13), shorter hospital stays and cost (10, 12, 13), and earlier recovery of function (14).

The case for setting up an effective orthoplastic service for the effective management of open long bone fractures is, therefore, compelling. The aim of this chapter is to describe how this can be achieved, the minimum required infrastructure for an operational orthoplastic unit, and to illustrate some of the systems and processes required in setting it up.

Requirements for the service

Initiating the model for change

There is no single model for effective implementation of a new service. Established practices are deep-rooted and may appear 'too difficult to' or 'not requiring' change. Every organisation will have its own approach to the delivery of patient care. The model for change is not an easy assignment. The ideal unit has to be aspired to, adequately resourced in terms of both clinical and managerial time, and the steps both owned and understood to enable service goals and outcomes to be achieved. The process should begin with engagement of senior management and consultants within the hospital trust or trusts. Clear leadership enables top-down commitment to delivering evidence-based practice. Having broken down the task into manageable stages, the approach to change can then be managed by 'incremental gains'.

Hospital set-up

There are three basic organisational structures that exist for the potential establishment of an orthoplastic unit within a major trauma network in England. First, there may be co-location of orthopaedic and plastic surgery (acute services) within the same hospital. The second scenario is that of cross-site working within the same trust. Finally, the two specialties may reside in different trusts. It goes without saying that the first situation is by far the most convenient for delivery of seamless care.

In a hospital with co-located services, the need for a new sub-specialty, driven clinically, is most likely to be supported at executive level if little infrastructural change is required. There is a potential for conflict between the specialties when funds are designated to a service not recognised as an income generator. However, the costs associated with the service can be recouped when the significant financial consequences of suboptimal management of open fractures are taken into consideration (15). The costs and income can then be shared equitably between specialties.

Cross-site working within the same trust is more challenging. Although trust objectives will be standardised across the hospitals, the move for part of the department to form the orthoplastic service at the site of the major trauma centre poses logistical challenges and additional investment will be required. Where plastic surgery services are not on site at the major trauma centre, this must be prioritised and capacity established for provision of a service that can provide free tissue transfer. This must be delivered by a group of consultants dedicated to ensure service provision every day of the week.

The most difficult circumstances for establishment of a new unit arise where services are in separate trusts. This is by far the most challenging set-up, as trusts face unique pressures and will have differing strategies to address these. There will be an even more significant burden for both cost and set-up. Even when executive-level support is achieved, the operational requirements, in terms of coordinating the services and the resources, management, administration, and information technology, will need financial and personal investment. A phased implementation plan may be required with a clear route to achieving key milestones and reviewed at regular intervals.

Whatever the structural organisation, it is imperative that there are dedicated leaders in both specialties for the orthoplastic unit to work. Furthermore, alongside the clinical expertise, there must be the infrastructure support for operational delivery of the service. Without this, there is an unsustainable scenario that will fail to deliver excellence in patient care. Irrespective of the precise model of the orthoplastic service, all institutions must share the same goal of providing combined care to the highest standards, as defined by national guidance (4, 5, 16, 17).

National support

Whilst Scotland, Wales, and Northern Ireland continue to develop their trauma provision, the most mature system in the UK is the major trauma network in England, with 26 major trauma centres. These provide an overall structure for trauma delivery, with support from surrounding trauma units and local emergency departments. These networks are supported by data collected via national reporting to the Trauma Audit Research Network (TARN). This allows each trauma network to assess and compare their delivery of major trauma care and continue to develop improvements towards the standards.

Local support

Each hospital trust must support the creation of the orthoplastic unit for provision of care for complex limb trauma. Executive- and board-level agreement is key. Local negotiations may take time and on occasion may appear fruitless, but the overriding agenda remains the provision of excellence in care for trauma as illustrated by the published standards (4, 16, 17). Alongside support within the hospital system, support from the local commissioning groups is also important. The major trauma and burns clinical reference group within NHS England produces the service specification. Centralised funding by way of specialist commissioning enables delivery of trauma care to be supported nationally. However, much complex orthoplastic limb reconstruction falls outside the national tariffs and support from local commissioners for a special local tariff can considerably enhance management support for service delivery.

Local commissioning

In order to recognise the 'front end' costs of the orthoplastic service for acute open fractures a meeting with local commissioners is essential. This will require detailed costing for the treatment of these patients in their current setting (18) to address the fiscal imbalance. These economic data can be presented together with audit data of patient numbers, demographics, and outcomes at the commissioners' meeting. This will enable the commissioners to evaluate the data and appreciate the cost-saving benefit of appropriately funding an effective orthoplastic service via agreed local tariffs.

Workforce planning

How many surgeons are required for an effective orthoplastic service? Is it feasible for every hospital in the UK treating open fractures to recruit several trauma-trained plastic surgeons to provide a microvascular service throughout the week and would the volume of work be sufficient to justify this? With crossover into other areas of plastic surgery sub-specialisation such as hand surgery, head and neck, or sarcoma, a plastic surgery department would likely have sufficient other complex cases to sustain a full orthoplastic service. The increasing numbers of open fragility fractures must also be factored in to service development.

If each of the 26 major trauma centres in England require six plastic surgeons for this service, then around 150 surgeons will be required nationally. Whilst this number may not sound daunting, there is no accurate information on plastic surgeons in practice or training with a special interest in trauma. Orthopaedic surgery has already seen a surge in interest in trauma as a career path and there are unlikely to be problems finding sufficient numbers of appropriately skilled surgeons in the future. Formal assessment of workforce and training needs would greatly assist workforce planning.

Working patterns in orthopaedics and plastic surgery need to provide consultant flexibility to perform open fracture wound excision with less than 12 hours' notice. The majority of these procedures would occur in daytime hours, so continuous daytime availability 7 days per week would be required, with an out-of-hours on-call facility. Whilst smaller units might struggle to achieve this, some larger departments have already moved to a consultant of the week or some other form of on-call arrangement where a consultant is available at all times to manage the unscheduled part of the service. Most NHS orthopaedic departments looking after major trauma have already developed this type of model.

The complexity of surgery for open fractures requires a dedicated all-day theatre list, with two or three such lists per week avoiding clashes with other plastic or orthopaedic surgery lists and the possibility of cancellation of elective cases. This would imply that two or three plastic and two or three orthopaedic surgeons are job-planned for those lists. Whilst this appears a significant commitment, it enables the strict timelines to be adhered to for the treatment of all open fractures.

No two hospitals in the NHS have the same working arrangements or on-call commitments for their orthopaedic or plastic surgeons. This suggests that there is no single ideal formula and local solutions need to be identified. However, those who are planning to provide a safe and effective orthoplastic service must have a degree of flexibility written and agreed in their job plans and dedicated sessions allocated for service provision.

Clinical involvement is not only restricted to dedicated consultant orthopaedic and plastic surgeons, available on call 24 hours a day, 7 days a week, but must also include other specialists such as infectious diseases/microbiology consultants, radiologists with specialist interest in musculoskeletal disorders, and rehabilitation consultants, together with allied healthcare professionals and specialist nurses. This multidisciplinary team must be supported by administrative assistance and fully coordinated so that continuous quality improvement is demonstrated.

Operational requirements

1) Facilities:
   - Access to trauma operating lists 24/7 for those fractures requiring immediate surgical intervention, such as the devascularised limb or the highly contaminated wound, or for return to theatre for a complication such as a compromised free flap.
   - Availability of combined operating lists for provision of definitive fixation and potential free flap coverage of open fractures during the week.
   - Weekly clinic for review.
   - Regular multidisciplinary team clinic with orthopaedic and plastic surgeons, physiotherapists, rehabilitation specialist, radiologist, microbiologist/infectious disease consultant.
   - Information technology support.

2) Personnel:
   - Plastic and orthopaedic consultant surgeons with a major commitment to trauma in their job plans and who can provide a full on-call service 24 hours a day, 7 days a week.
   - Specialist nursing teams on the ward who have the skills to care for the complex trauma patient from both an orthopaedic and plastic surgery perspective, in particular with reference to managing the postoperative course for both plastic surgery free tissue transfer and orthopaedic circular frames, external fixators, and pin sites.
   - Consultant microbiologist.
   - Specialist theatre staff for orthopaedic fixation and free flap surgery.
   - Outpatient nursing for dressings.
   - Plaster technicians and orthotic expertise.
   - Physiotherapists for mobilisation and care of the polytrauma patient.
   - Rehabilitation expertise with reference to amputation and prosthetic requirements.
   - Consultant rehabilitation specialists.
   - Dedicated administrative support.
   - Dedicated service management support.
   - A dedicated coordinator to support the case management of patients.

Cost effectiveness

The true cost of trauma is unknown. The financial costs of immediate trauma care have been estimated at between £0.3 and £0.4 billion a year (19). Costs for subsequent hospital treatments, rehabilitation, social care home support, and individual personal care are difficult to calculate, and the cost to an individual in terms of function and loss of earnings are undetermined. Figures from the National Audit Office estimate a lost annual economic output of up to £3.7 billion.

A robust systems approach was adopted by the NICE Guidance Development Groups regarding clinical evidence and cost effectiveness. Cost effectiveness denotes the expected costs of different options in relation to their expected health benefit, rather than total implementation cost (20). The available data were reviewed and modelled by health economists at NICE.

The cost efficacy for the combined orthoplastic approach for the treatment of open fractures for patients managed at specialist centres was elegantly demonstrated (4). Sequential care by plastic surgeons following initial orthopaedic management was associated with higher infection rates, increased numbers of surgical procedures and inter-hospital transfers for non-co-located specialties, and prolonged hospital stay dramatically increased the cost per patient.

NICE considered the evidence relating to the presence of the plastic surgeon with the orthopaedic surgeon at the initial surgical wound excision and stabilisation. This was split into three areas: the initial wound excision, the timing of soft tissue cover, and potential multiple theatre sessions. Various outcome measures were considered, including unplanned complexity of the soft tissue reconstruction (impacting on surgical time, equipment, and staffing), free flap failure, as well as hospital stay and further unplanned surgery. The results demonstrated a reduction in the costs associated with wound excision at all time points if a plastic surgeon was present. This is because, even with the additional staff and theatre time, the combined orthoplastic approach resulted in fewer complications and hence was cost effective.

Other clinical studies have investigated comparisons between treatment between the two specialties and that combined in one unit. Specifically considering healthcare utilisation, Page et al. demonstrated that when patients with open tibial fractures were admitted directly to an orthoplastic centre, they had significantly fewer operations and GP attendances thereafter, compared with patients undergoing initial management elsewhere, with subsequent transfer (21).

Whilst the cost and clinical benefits are compelling, the initial investment required to set up the service can be extremely challenging.

So how do you do it?

The NICE guidance and quality standards can be used as levers to implement change and introduce best working practices to achieve optimal patient outcomes. The optimum route to growing a service will depend on the environment. Successful orthoplastic units in England have grown their service progressively (7, 18). This perspective from cross-trust working in the UK has led us to consider the stepwise approach when clinical priorities must be balanced alongside financial and care quality pressures.

- Short, medium, and long-term goals must be established and the availability of limited resources recognised.

- Executive support is key to sponsoring and ensuring the release of management and clinical time and other resources.

- Board member appreciation of the goal to provide excellent patient care in line with national guidance.

- With any collaborative board set-up, central representation from NHS England or equivalent is also required and important so all commissioners are represented.

- If financial pressures or trust directives become more of a priority, the negotiations for orthoplastic capacity should centre on NICE quality standards and guidance.

- This requires alignment of the trust(s) strategic objectives with provision of excellent patient care, and the potential for changes within departments, such as addition of staff members, separate business cases that will support not only the case for trauma but more generic need on wards, clinics, and in theatres.

- Utilise the major trauma peer review process and GIRFT (get it right first time) reviews for plastics and orthopaedic trauma to benchmark progress and facilitate change.

- Engage those other departments and directorates that have both a key interest and dependency on the service and where an essential partnership and joint working is needed.

- Raise the risk of the service to the trust for risk register reporting if the service is not appropriately resourced or where patient care may be compromised.

- Represent the unit nationally at association trauma interest groups and national trauma meetings.

- Major trauma networks and clinical governance reporting will continue to raise the agenda nationally to the major trauma clinical directorate and TARN.

- Outcomes and audit must continue to be presented departmentally, hospital-wide, regionally, and nationally, together with publications.

Conclusion

This chapter aims to give insight into the most important prerequisite for the delivery of the Standards: that of the orthoplastic unit. The merits of this set-up have been recognised worldwide, and yet, in the cost-pressured NHS we are yet to achieve this gold standard in all of our major trauma centres throughout England and the rest of the UK.

We have defined what is required, and highlighted the evidence for the need for this combined management. We have highlighted the difficulties encountered. It can take 5 years or more to achieve this standard of care. Delivering optimal outcomes in terms of a functional limb and a rehabilitated patient in a cost-efficient manner remains at the heart of service development and delivery.

References

1. **Court-Brown CM, Rimmer S, Prakash U, McQueen MM.** The epidemiology of open long bone fractures. Injury. 1998;**29**(7):529–34.
2. **Court-Brown CM, Biant LC, Clement ND, Bugler KE, Duckworth AD, McQueen MM.** Open fractures in the elderly. The importance of skin ageing. Injury. 2015;**46**(2):189–94.
3. **Court-Brown CM, Bugler KE, Clement ND, Duckworth AD, McQueen MM.** The epidemiology of open fractures in adults. A 15-year review. Injury. 2012;**43**(6):891–7.
4. **National Clinical Guideline Centre (UK).** Fractures (Complex): Assessment and Management. London: National Institute for Health and Care Excellence (UK); 2016 Feb. NG37. https://www.nice.org.uk/guidance/ng37/chapter/Recommendations#hospital-settings
5. **National Institute for Health and Care Excellence.** Major Trauma: Service Delivery NICE Guideline (NG40). London: National Institute for Health and Care Excellence (UK); 2016.
6. **National Institute for Health and Care Excellence.** Quality Standard for Trauma [QS166]. London: National Institute for Health and Care Excellence (UK); 2018.
7. **Mathews JA, Ward J, Chapman TW, Khan UM, Kelly MB.** Single-stage orthoplastic reconstruction of Gustilo-Anderson Grade III open tibial fractures greatly reduces infection rates. Injury. 2015;**46**(11):2263–6.
8. **Ali AM, McMaster JM, Noyes D, Brent AJ, Cogswell LK.** Experience of managing open fractures of the lower limb at a major trauma centre. Ann R Coll Surg Engl. 2015;**97**(4):287–90.
9. **Chummun S, Wright TC, Chapman TW, Khan U.** Outcome of the management of open ankle fractures in an ortho-plastic specialist centre. Injury. 2015;**46**(6):1112–15.
10. **Sommar P, Granberg Y, Halle M, Skogh AC, Lundgren KT, Jansson KA.** Effects of a formalized collaboration between plastic and orthopedic surgeons in severe extremity trauma patients; a retrospective study. J Trauma Manag Outcomes. 2015;**9**:3.
11. **Trickett RW, Rahman S, Page P, Pallister I.** From guidelines to standards of care for open tibial fractures. Ann R Coll Surg Engl. 2015;**97**(6):469–75.

12. Fernandez MA, Wallis K, Venus M, Skillman J, Young J, Costa ML. The impact of a dedicated orthoplastic operating list on time to soft tissue coverage of open lower limb fractures. Ann R Coll Surg Engl. 2015;97(6):456–9.

13. Sargazi N, El-Gawad A, Narayan B, Bell D, Shanks L, Nayagam S, et al. A full time regional ortho-plastic unit; initial results. JPRAS. 2016;69(4):572–3.

14. Boriani F, Ul Haq A, Baldini T, Urso R, Granchi D, Baldini N, et al. Orthoplastic surgical collaboration is required to optimise the treatment of severe limb injuries: a multi-centre, prospective cohort study. JPRAS. 2017;70(6):715–22.

15. Tissingh EK, Memarzadeh A, Queally J, Hull P. Open lower limb fractures in major trauma centers—a loss leader? Injury. 2017;48(2):353–6.

16. British Orthopaedic Association. British Association of Plastic, Reconstructive and Aesthetic Surgeons. Audit Standards for Trauma: Open Fractures. London: BOA; 2017.

17. Nanchahal J, Nayagam S, Khan U, Moran C, Barrett S, Sanderson F, et al. Standards for the Management of Open Fractures of the Lower Limb. London: BAPRAS; 2009.

18. Townley WA, Urbanska C, Dunn RL, Khan U. Costs and coding—free-flap reconstruction in lower-limb trauma. Injury. 2011;42(4):381–4.

19. National Audit Office. Major Trauma Care in England. London: NAO; 2010.

20. National Institute for Health and Care Excellence. The Guidelines Manual. London: NICE; 2012.

21. Page PR, Trickett RW, Rahman SM, Walters A, Pinder LM, Brooks CJ, et al. The use of secure anonymised data linkage to determine changes in healthcare utilisation following severe open tibial fractures. Injury. 2015;46(7):1287–92.

Chapter 21

NICE Recommendations Relevant to Open Fractures

Introduction

In 2016 the National Institute for Clinical and Care Excellence (NICE) published a suite of five trauma-related guidelines including the Guideline on Complex Fractures NG37. A significant component of this guideline related specifically to open fractures. Following the publication of that complete trauma suite of five related guidelines there was further work by NICE resulting in the formulation of a Quality Standard Statement. A NICE quality standard is a concise set of statements designed to drive and measure priority quality improvements within a particular area of care. For the entire trauma suite this was distilled to five statements; one of these was specific to open fractures.

The relevant recommendations from the NICE guideline NG37 and statement from the Quality Standard are included and presented below both for easy reference. It also allows the concordance that exists between the text in the rest of this book, the Open Fracture BOAST and NICE to be better appreciated.

© NICE (2016) NG37 Fractures (Complex): Assessment and Management. Available from www.nice.org.uk/guidance/ng37 All rights reserved. Subject to Notice of rights.

NICE guidance is prepared for the National Health Service in England. All NICE guidance is subject to regular review and may be updated or withdrawn. NICE accepts no responsibility for the use of its content in this product/ publication.

Quality Standards—QS166

Statement 3 People with open fractures of long bones, the hindfoot or midfoot have fixation and definitive soft tissue cover within 72 hours of injury if this cannot be performed at the same time as debridement.

Extracts from NICE recommendations Complex Fractures NG37 2016

1.1 Pre-hospital settings

Initial management of open fractures before debridement

1.1.8 Do not irrigate open fractures of the long bones, hindfoot or midfoot in pre-hospital settings.

1.1.9 Consider a saline-soaked dressing covered with an occlusive layer for open fractures in pre-hospital settings.

1.1.10 In the pre-hospital setting, consider administering prophylactic intravenous antibiotics as soon as possible and preferably within 1 hour of injury to people with open fractures without delaying transport to hospital.

Splinting long bone fractures of the leg in the pre-hospital setting

1.1.11 In the pre-hospital setting, consider the following for people with suspected long bone fractures of the legs:

- a traction splint or adjacent leg as a splint if the suspected fracture is above the knee
- a vacuum splint for all other suspected long bone fractures.

Destination for people with suspected fractures

1.1.12 Transport people with suspected open fractures:

- directly to a major trauma centre or specialist centre that can provide orthoplastic care if a long bone, hindfoot or midfoot are involved, or
- to the nearest trauma unit or emergency department if the suspected fracture is in the hand, wrist or toes, unless there are pre-hospital triage indications for direct transport to a major trauma centre.

1.2 Hospital settings

Vascular injury

1.2.1 Use hard signs (lack of palpable pulse, continued blood loss, or expanding haematoma) to diagnose vascular injury.

1.2.2 Do not rely on capillary return or Doppler signal to exclude vascular injury.

1.2.3 Perform immediate surgical exploration if hard signs of vascular injury persist after any necessary restoration of limb alignment and joint reduction.

1.2.4 In people with a devascularised limb following long bone fracture, use a vascular shunt as the first surgical intervention before skeletal stabilisation and definitive vascular reconstruction.

1.2.5 Do not delay revascularisation for angiography in people with complex fractures.

Whole-body CT of multiple injuries

1.2.8 Use whole-body CT (consisting of a vertex-to-toes scanogram followed by CT from vertex to mid-thigh) in adults (16 or over) with blunt major trauma and suspected multiple injuries. Patients should not be repositioned during whole-body CT.

1.2.9 Use clinical findings and the scanogram to direct CT of the limbs in adults (16 or over) with limb trauma.

Management of open fractures before debridement

1.2.20 Do not irrigate open fractures of the long bones, hindfoot or midfoot in the emergency department before debridement.

1.2.21 Consider a saline-soaked dressing covered with an occlusive layer (if not already applied) for open fractures in the emergency department before debridement.

1.2.22 In the emergency department, administer prophylactic intravenous antibiotics immediately to people with open fractures if not already given.

Limb salvage in people with open fractures

1.2.23 Do not base the decision whether to perform limb salvage or amputation on an injury severity tool score.

1.2.24 Perform emergency amputation when:

- a limb is the source of uncontrollable life-threatening bleeding, or
- a limb is salvageable but attempted preservation would pose an unacceptable risk to the person's life, or
- a limb is deemed unsalvageable after orthoplastic assessment.

Include the person and their family members or carers (as appropriate) in a full discussion of the options if this is possible.

1.2.25 Base the decision whether to perform limb salvage or delayed primary amputation on multidisciplinary assessment involving an orthopaedic surgeon, a plastic surgeon, a rehabilitation specialist and the person and their family members or carers (as appropriate).

1.2.26 When indicated, perform the delayed primary amputation within 72 hours of injury.

Debridement, staging of fixation and cover

1.2.27 Surgery to achieve debridement, fixation and cover of open fractures of the long bone, hindfoot or midfoot should be performed concurrently by consultants in orthopaedic and plastic surgery (a combined orthoplastic approach).

1.2.28 Perform debridement:

- immediately for highly contaminated open fractures
- within 12 hours of injury for high-energy open fractures (likely Gustilo–Anderson classification type IIIA or type IIIB) that are not highly contaminated
- within 24 hours of injury for all other open fractures.

1.2.29 Perform fixation and definitive soft tissue cover:

- at the same time as debridement if the next orthoplastic list allows this within the time to debridement recommended in 1.2.28, or
- within 72 hours of injury if definitive soft tissue cover cannot be performed at the time of debridement.

1.2.30 When internal fixation is used, perform definitive soft tissue cover at the same time.

1.3 **Documentation**

Photographic documentation of open fracture wounds

1.3.4 All trusts receiving patients with open fractures must have information governance policies in place that enable staff to take and use photographs of open fracture wounds for clinical decision-making 24 hours a day. Protocols must also cover the handling and storage of photographic images of open fracture wounds.

1.3.5 Consider photographing open fracture wounds when they are first exposed for clinical care, before debridement and at other key stages of management.

1.3.6 Keep any photographs of open fracture wounds in the patient's records.

Documentation of neurovascular status

1.3.7 When assessing neurovascular status in a person with a limb injury, document for both limbs:

- which nerves and nerve function have been assessed and when

- the findings, including:
  - sensibility
  - motor function using the Medical Research Council (MRC) grading system
- which pulses have been assessed and when
- how circulation has been assessed when pulses are not accessible.

Document and time each repeated assessment.

1.5 **Training and skills**

These recommendations are for ambulance and hospital trust boards, medical directors and senior managers within trauma networks

1.5.1 Ensure that each healthcare professional within the trauma service has the training and skills to deliver, safely and effectively, the interventions they are required to give, in line with the NICE guidelines on non-complex fractures, complex fractures, major trauma, major trauma services and spinal injury assessment.

1.5.2 Enable each healthcare professional who delivers care to people with fractures to have up-to-date training in the interventions they are required to give.

Index

Tables and boxed material appear in **bold**; figures in *italic* following the page number.

For the benefit of digital users, indexed terms that span two pages (e.g., 52–53) may, on occasion, appear on only one of those pages.